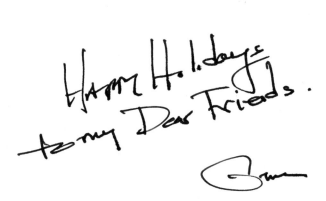

Happy Holidays
to my Dear Friends.

WHAT
2
WHY

Eugene Keller, MD, MBA

TABLE OF CONTENTS

ISBN: 978-1-66787-521-7 print

ISBN: 978-1-66786-415-0 ebook

I.
PREFACE

In many ways, I have been a part of a period in medicine that rivals the introduction of sterile technique and anesthesia over a century ago. Those breakthroughs altered the course of patient care and how we, as caregivers, related to our patients. Several internal and external factors have indelibly changed modern medicine in many subtle and less publicized ways.

Overall, health and the response to disease have improved dramatically owing to technological advances, expanded research capabilities, information distribution, and safety measures. The cost of medical care has surged disproportionally in our economy, and with it has come increasing control by governmental and financially motivated organizations. Much of this has been at least partially responsible for the disruption of the relationship between the caregiver and the patient. The advanced technologies, as currently deployed, stand stolidly between human contact and have terminally altered the personal relationship between the doctor, caregivers of all types, and the patient.

In what follows, I have attempted to bring together my thoughts and have included insights from multiple experts in medicine and related fields. This allows for a better appreciation of our current status in medicine, primarily in the United States. After achieving a better, honest understanding, I have included suggestions and pathways of how we, as caregivers and those needing care, can adjust, perhaps even slightly, how we do things and incorporate where we are and where we need to be.

I have participated in many exciting and rewarding efforts in my years in the field. Cracking the chest (emergency thoracotomy) of a sixteen-year-old with a stab wound to the heart, emergently inserting my finger in the myocardium's traumatic hole, and saving the patient's life was pretty special. Perhaps surprisingly, participating in system improvements, working side by side with physicians, nurses, and the rest of the care teams, which have impacted the safety and quality of care for tens of thousands of patients, has had a distinct satisfaction.

In the "old days," we were told that, if we had appropriate verifiable data on how we were doing, publishing that information would significantly improve what and how we did things, specifically in the quality and safety of patient care. This is absolute truth but only to a degree. Using the overwhelming data that is increasingly available to actualize our goals continues to be a labor of love.

Peppered throughout this work are many case studies that I sincerely hope personalize at some level the material within. The cases are pretty accurate, but the specific patients they represent are not.

When asked originally, as I started this writing task, to whom might this book be of interest, I was unsure of my potential audience. I believe there are some insights and even conclusions, despite my biases, that could serve as reminders to those of us in the field of what is our ultimate goal.

However, I think that the general public could also find this material quite pertinent to their daily lives, not only as it sheds insights into our current medical system, but how engagement, personal responsibility, and accountability are the basis of successful systems of all types.

Much of the material contained within the book is based on my career as a practicing emergency physician and a health care executive. However, when reading over the material, I discovered that many lessons applied to non-medical settings. It may seem obvious that the core connection between the patient and caregiver in medicine is essential, but in practice, this is less and less so. There is also no presumption that this connection is necessary for more automated fields outside of patient care activities.

The title of this book represents that the focus for many organizations, including health care, is on WHAT is happening. We now have reams of available data reflective of what we do daily, weekly, etc. What we do with that information depends on the WHY things happen, which requires dedicated analysis. These two W words encompass a great deal of discussion within the Five Ws of this book: WHAT2WHY2WHAT2WHY2WHAT.

Each W has its section, but as you shall see, there is a considerable cross-over, and each section helps modify those around it.

My goal has always been to empower all elements of the complicated care web and galvanize caregivers and patients and their families to truly take a more active role in all aspects of their health.

II.
INTRODUCTION

It was pretty dark in the cave and the air was filled with smoke and ash. The flickering minimal light shed by the dwindling fire did not reach the bodies clustered in its far reaches. An occasional movement or murmur was lost to the sound of moaning that pierced the smoke-filled blackness. Closer to the white coals at the fire pit base lay a single figure, clad in an oily hide covering only his genitals, holding his arm up in a pleading gesture. Blackened fingernails protruded from a scabbed and filthy hand. He pointed to his abdomen and looked at the men squatting around him with frantic eyes. Their voices raised as the figure cried out and drew his knees to his chest.

Moments later, a shadow pierced the dim light coming from the mouth of the cave. Indistinct but wearing a headdress topped with skins and antlers, the figure moved toward the group clustered around the prone body by the fire. Guttural sounds of greeting followed him as he moved forward. He kneeled carefully on the stone floor. Minimal words were spoken, and the figure adorned with animal skins threw stained and worn animal bones on the cave floor from a leather sack he pulled from around his neck. He studied the pattern of bones, making repeated animal-like barking sounds as he did so, beseeching the spirits. He then suddenly shifted his gaze to the prone figure near the fire. The clustered men halted their movement and watched as the heavily adorned newcomer reached out his hand and gently touched the suffering man. The medicine man prodded the lying man's abdomen with troubled eyes and was rewarded with writhing and moaning.

The first history of men who joined together in the struggle against disease was recorded by Cro-Magnon artists about twenty thousand years ago. Evidence discovered in caves in Dordogne, France, was the first record of a doctor as there had been no written or pictorial language. In Ariege France, a particular cave contained actual grease paint pictures of the first prehistoric representation of a medicine man. The use of grease in the paint has helped preserve the colors from the moist air and water over the millenniums (1).

It should be noted from the suffering man on the floor of the cave that the ritual reading of bones was the primary diagnostic approach. Yet, in this instance, the medicine man redefined his role by reaching out and touching the patient. He confirmed a bond with that physical contact and tactilely added to his understanding of the patient's underlying condition. Even though twenty thousand years ago there was no help for the "patient" that would soon die from a ruptured appendix, he took halting first steps on a path that would morph into modern medicine.

These early healing practitioners were predominantly translators of spirits, religion, and magic while touching those suffering from disease and trauma. It was not until Hippocrates that medicine started to rise out of the veil of mysticism and belief. Although considered the father of medicine, it was not for his abilities as a doctor to cure but his interest in facts that propelled us forward. He attempted to define the difference between the sick and the well, and "he scrutinized sick men and recorded honesty the signs and symptoms of disease honestly theorizing" [(2) p. 65].

It is perhaps him that we have to thank for the journey of embracing knowledge and facts to advance the safety and quality of the patients we serve. Yet, it should be noted that we are still on this trek. Unfortunately, we are still struggling despite generations of medical professionals, scientists, academics, and even the advent of the computer and its ramifications.

Multiple advances in medical technology and laboratory medicine have raised the bar in inpatient care, but untoward events and medical mishaps occur daily. There are numerous factors for this situation, gleefully reported in various modern lay communications, that yearly cause hundreds of thousands of medical errors and associated deaths. These factors must be put in a statistical perspective. Nevertheless, a single medical error or substandard care for any patient is an anathema to what we hold most dear to us. As physicians, our personal goal has always been to care for our patients every single day. We have humbly recognized the ownership of that duty and the accountability it represents.

This book represents efforts to understand the state of modern medicine, discuss how we got here, and not criticize our colleagues or those who have come before us. I know the fantastic resources in our world and hope to present some clues on how best to utilize what is available and envision our future and how to "get there." Some of the "stories" are taken from personal experience; some are compilations, and some are gleaned from the experiences of others, either from direct communication or from the literature.

As you engage with this material, you will find many themes that play through the specific discussions on the subsequent pages. They reflect firmly held opinions, and perhaps even selected references have been cited. Danial Kahneman would suggest that we, like most everyone, have our *biases* (3). He and Amos Tversky virtually invented the field of behavioral economics. Still, their material is exceptionally pertinent to how we make decisions in medicine, not just in the large-scale system and data issues, but at the bedside, taking care of a single patient. Their understanding of heuristics in multiple papers led to Kahneman winning the Nobel Prize after Tversky's death. In evaluating decisions, the theme of bias is one of the elements woven into the discussions in later pages. I will openly discuss my own biases and some of the reasons for writing this book.

Perhaps the first bias that does not even have a chapter or section devoted to it is that we can never overlook that medicine has been and always should be about basic humanity. It is ultimately people taking care of people. The essential tableau of the medicine man in the cave was his reaching out to touch the sick man, not his crying out to the spirits, not his belief in the bones, but in the confluence of his life with that of his patient. As a physician, the outstretched hand of the medicine man, the human touch, so much symbolized one of the critical elements in caring for patients.

The physician or APP (advanced care provider) of today has multiple arrows in their quiver for both the diagnosis and treatment of the patient. The introduction of the electronic health record (EHR) and the fundamental belief in its Artificial Intelligence (more accurately automated intelligence or assisted intelligence) has distracted, at least in part, the doctor's focus from the bedside. The average provider spends significantly more time ordering and evaluating information from various sources, such as lab, radiology, MRI, and cardiac catheterizations, than with the patient. Add to this the time spent in the laborious documentation now demanded by the EHR; it is no wonder that patients don't know who their provider is. This too will be a theme in the following pages.

As with society in general, medicine is changing extremely rapidly. Writing this during the Covid-19 pandemic highlights some of the external forces that merge with the internal influences that offer opportunities for change and demand a rapid adaption that few of us are used to. A few years ago, the diligent care provider would read the medical journals delivered to his door. Getting something written and then published was a rigorous process that took months or even years. The Internet has obliterated this lengthy process, and we now see articles and scientific data presented almost daily that record information and discoveries from just yesterday. Although an excellent source for keeping providers up-to-date, there is so much information that selectivity trumps literacy in wide-ranging areas. A practitioner felt pretty good if he kept up with two or three publications directed in his specialty. Now the information stream is so vast that, to stay current, the priorities of the modern provider demand a narrower scope. This favors specialists who can focus on new information in limited and more biased fields.

This trend in specialization has participated in significant advances in medical therapeutics and outcomes but has somewhat complicated the continuity of patient care in our health care system. Factor in the popularity of hospitalists, and the average number of individual physicians seeing a patient during a single stay in today's hospital is three and one half. The concept of physicians wholly committed to taking care of only hospitalized patients is not new. Training programs for physicians now focus on preparing doctors to focus on patients meeting the criteria for hospitalization. Hospitalists are on-site, many twenty-four hours a day, seven days a week. For the most part, nurses calling doctors in their offices to react to rapid changes in sick patients or the response to results of a myriad of testing has been replaced with this onsite shift coverage of dedicated, well-trained in-house practitioners. However, owing to the diversity of treating individuals and the pull of the provider by the EHR (Electronic Health Record), many patients, when asked who their doctor is, cannot identify them.

Procuring follow-up care for patients discharged from the hospital continues to be a significant problem. Seeing their own primary care physician after an inpatient stay is far from a slam dunk. Because of its issues, continuity of care, both in the inpatient and outpatient setting, will be another leitmotif in the following chapters. There are medical systems where continuity of care is a priority, both from the quality and financial drivers, but this is still not the rule across hospitals and health care systems.

The EHR (Electronic Health Record) advent was dedicated to supporting continuity of care. Sharing in-depth information about a patient on multiple platforms significantly enhances communication between medical providers and nurses, techs, respiratory therapists, physical therapists, social workers, and care coordinators in the hospital and outpatient offices and facilities. When this works well, it certainly provides in-depth information in a very timely manner. Still, it is dependent on often laborious and time-consuming computer-based documentation by the folks mentioned above.

The other focus of EHR is patient safety. Built-in prompts, safety measures, and care plans, for example, help providers not make mistakes but have complicated patient care. There is an internal struggle between too much and too little in EHR that may delay and compromise overall responses to rapidly changing and complex patient issues.

The good, the bad, and the ugly of our integration of the EHR, I hope, will not be a primary theme of this book, although based on our experiences, it may sneak in as part of my bias.

The elements of culture and leadership are essential to stand up. From my experience in multiple medical organizations, I hope the concepts, tools, and plans in the following pages will help providers move steadily toward safety and patient care quality. There will be in-depth conversations, but it is essential to understand the importance of the medical milieu. I will try to define the leadership and culture necessary for an organization to achieve lofty goals overall and in the care of every patient.

The book's title "WHAT2WHY" is one of several "alphabetical" usage techniques to allow readers to hold on to concepts for discussion, thoughts, and mastery.

WHAT2WHY2WHAT2 WHY2WHAT

The five **W**s each will have its section, but they are also thematic throughout the book. Many things can impact the safety and quality of patient care within our medical system. The first and perhaps foremost of these is an understanding of **WHAT** is our business. This is the makeup of our organization's culture, leadership, and goals. The second **W**, or **WHY**, is a question about the internal makeup of the people who inhabit the medical community themselves. What are their backgrounds, beliefs, hopes, and dreams, and where are they in their development? It tries to answer **WHY** am I here and provide an understanding of the elements of their personal and professional lives. There will be a lot of discussion about processes and outcomes, but we are in a people business, and we are internally setting the stage for our perspective

After receiving her doctorate from Harvard University and teaching at George Mason University, Jennifer Garvey Berger, in her book <u>Changing on the Job</u> (4), discusses the understanding of perspectives, one's own and that of others, as a critical feature in **WHY** I am here. It also highlights a bit of a sense of how their perspectives mitigate the **WHAT** of our leaders. "Taking multiple perspectives enables people to see a wider range of possibilities, make deeper connections, and understand the views of others . . . One key to transformational and sustainable professional development is the degree to which taking multiple perspectives becomes a habit" (5).

Framing, or reframing based on inputs becomes a critical attribute in the balance of **WHY** we are here. Sam Sommers in his book <u>Situations Matter,</u> points out; "So much of what we see and interact with the social universe around us is shaped by our immediate context. Seemingly trivial aspects of daily situations determine whether to keep to ourselves or get involved in affairs of others…" (6)

One of our emergency physicians was having a run of complaints about his care from patients. I reviewed the medical records carefully and only found exceptional technical evaluations, decision-making, and outcomes. Phone calls to some of the patients who had complained revealed many observations and issues about the young doctor. Still, at first, the underlying theme of the patients' dissatisfaction was difficult to ascertain. An older female patient finally said, "He doesn't seem to care." This is an unusual but not unheard-of complaint in busy emergency departments throughout the United States. The ER doctor may be running between ten to fifteen patients at a time, with a wide variety of urgencies and true emergencies, barely able to spend a few minutes with each patient. These complaints have not caused me to remember the situation but the doctor's response as I discussed it. "The patients feel that you don't care," I said. He turned to me, looked me squared in the face, and said, "I don't really. I am an excellent clinician, don't make mistakes, haven't been sued, and do my job!"

Subsequently, we had many conversations about the **WANT** of his **WHY**, which further elucidated his perspectives and personal development and would mitigate his role moving forward. Most times, the evidence of what people *want* is buried in complex relationships, job duties, and social development. It is rarely factored into discussing what hard data is telling us.

As the coming chapters unfold and we discuss the increasing amount of medical data available for analysis and action, we want to keep the role of people constantly in focus. When we look at the part of the "culture "of a hospital or medical organization, individuals with leadership roles may view data differently on the basis of their inner mantra. Although my experience is primarily from medical situations, I believe that the participation of the individual and what they think about themselves is transcendental in how they perform within most other structured organizations.

Let's venture into the complex world of how to provide the highest level of quality and safety and comfort for our patients.

In this discussion of **WHAT** we are as an organization and **WHY** we are here as individuals, we cannot forget the patient's *WANTS*. Our caveman would probably have wanted only to be relieved of pain. Patients today have a sometimes-unfulfillable expectation of what modern medicine can do. This is imposed on us, in many ways, by the technological marvels that now grace the armamentarium of the contemporary practitioner. The presumption of an immediate diagnosis, or at least the relief of symptoms, is somewhat deserved as our diagnostic and therapeutic capabilities improve yearly. However, the relentless advertisements about the breadth and extent of medications can't help but point the suffering patient to a place where the alleviation of all symptoms, if not a cure, is not only possible but probable.

The **WHAT** we are about is often focused on the financial aspects of care no matter how ecumenical *what* we *want* is. The profitability of pharmaceutical options, the need to constantly update medical equipment, the cost of implantable devices, and escalating personnel salaries are severe deterrents to controlling rising healthcare costs. Health care systems may position themselves with quite laudable goals. Still, the pressure on the bottom line puts a tremendous squeeze on the purest motivation of **WHAT** we are as an organization.

Finances play a significant role in the **WHY** we as individuals are here. But from my years of experience, it was job satisfaction, the attachment to peers and teams, and self-fulfillment that provided the most significant rewards.

The third **W** is **WHAT**, which stands for what we know. Admittedly the integration of computerized systems into health care has expanded the depth and breadth of available information about what we do. For decades, because of the variability of patients and their illnesses, the measure of quality and safe care was often solely in the practitioner's mind. Even when accurate data was presented, the lack of controls and statistically tested values had us evert to define good care in our image. "My patients are sicker" was the common refrain when numbers for an individual physician seemed to point to problems or the need for improvement. Today's data is timely, statistically significant, and gives us insight into **WHAT** we are doing daily. Numbers or percentages often judge today's quality care and the safety of care reflects the numerical demonstration of "zero harm."

A more detailed discussion, perhaps too elaborate, about the third **WHAT** comes later in this work.

As part of elucidating the elements of **WHAT** (the first **WHAT**), understanding an organization's culture of safety and quality is imperative.

In defining what we are, Edgar Shein (7), a world-renowned expert on organizational culture and credited with founding the field, in his book *Organizational Culture and leadership,* describes culture as follows:

- Observed behavioral regularities

- Climate, the feelings conveyed in a group, and the way members interact

- Formal rituals and celebrations

- Espoused values, group norms and standards

- Identity and image of self

- Shared meanings or commonality of language

- I would add one more essential element of culture: resource management and allocation. Posting the goals in the main lobby needs to reflect the commitment of time and resources and finances to achieving those goals. "Put your money where your mouth is" is an old saying central to success and achieving a culture of trust in an organization.

In hospitals or health care systems, some of the most visible manifestations of culture are the overtly published and featured goals, the demonstrated executive and management leadership, the functionality of teams, and quality and safety. One can gain a gestalt feeling of these elements, but in the health care field, quality and safety, being the most important, are probably the most easily measurable.

As with many organizations inside and outside the medical world, safety and quality, as interpreted through increasingly available data, have become a primary building block of **WHAT** an organization is and how it is represented.

We argue a lot about whether it is quality or safety, and the copious data that now comes from the study of each is the lynchpin in understanding excellent patient care. In some discussions, quality and safety are portrayed as overlapping circles.

In general terms, of course, we want all patients under all circumstances to have the safest quality-driven experience. But what does that mean? The language of safety has become increasingly specific over the last decade, and a vast amount of published data and discussion has followed. Owing to unheeded warnings about the O rings, the Shuttle disaster had added fuel to the reports of hundreds of thousands of lives lost because of medical errors. Patient names and children's photos now pepper the lay press, and the discussion of safety in hospitals is often the talk of national news and forums.

Attention in the medical field about safety has been discussed for decades. It was not until the nineties that a published report from the Institute of Medicine (IOM) called "To Err is Human" started to galvanize a more aggressive approach to patient safety. In addition, two widely publicized pediatric cases, Libby Zion and Emily Jerry, and the punitive and financial penalties attributable to those cases, caused an outpouring of public sentiment. Subsequently, hospitals, which had been the main focus of this attention, have added personnel and programs to react to these safety issues. Unfortunately, continued monitoring shows that there has been less than a significant statistical impact on nationally reported mortality numbers (8).

This is not equally true with our quality numbers, which have shown a continual slow improvement. An example of this is the mortality numbers for severe sepsis, which have continued to decline over the last decade. Is this a fact, or is it an example of the definition and measurement differences between these two closely monitored indices? Severe sepsis and the vigorous campaign for its early recognition and treatment fill many academic journals and are also a standing discussion in the boardrooms of most hospitals.

It isn't easy, as mentioned, to separate the concepts of safety and quality since there is considerable overlap in the application, the measurement, and the tools for the assessment of these mandates. For the most part, organizations such as IHI (Institute of Healthcare Improvement), consulting with hospitals in developing HRO (high-reliability organizations), utilize technology to track *errors* that produce "harm" events (9). They use programs such as IVOS (incident reporting system) and RTM (risk trigger monitoring) to look for individual events, from a safety perspective, that potentially have serious complications from errors.

The incident reporting system or hospital-specific organizational name relies on staff reporting events that meet specific criteria, like a retained foreign body and if the staff "feels" it does not meet safety expectations. Staff routinely enter specific data into the computerized health information system, which has a well-developed, choreographed response from the hospital leadership. There is wide variability in reporting, mitigated by the organizations' culture and sensitivity to process and outcome. Almost all data about IVOS programs recognize a tremendous amount of underreporting.

RTM (Root Trigger Monitoring) is a process supplied by Pascal Metrics that scans the EHR records every fifteen minutes and looks for eighty different "triggers" associated with errors or poor outcomes. For example, opioids given to patients after surgical or interventional procedures are looked at very carefully. Suppose a patient, particularly with risk factors, has an order for a dose of medication that might develop problems such as respiratory distress. In that case, RTM triggers a response that can significantly alter the patient's care after the screening. IVOS only reports about 20 percent of those triggers automatically reported by RTM in our facilities.

When RTM is appropriately resourced, and staff is assigned to react to RTM reports, there is an opportunity to stop or reverse, or at least concurrently respond to, a potential individual patient risk issue. This data is then collated and used for education and process improvement. IVOS and similar programs also add much to staff education and PI (process improvement), but it is only retrospective and rarely impacts immediate patient care. Both programs facilitate organizational commitment to notify patients and families immediately of any potential safety issues or deviations from accepted standard practice. This is a critical factor in the culture of an organization. Full disclosure and timely communication with patients are essential at every leadership level and among clinical personnel, no matter the issue.

Mishaps, reported and validated by RTM and IVOS, are usually studied in depth by a process called event analysis or an RCA (root cause analysis). RCA is not unique to medical organizations but appears in multiple forms throughout many industries. The medical field, particularly the hospital world, brings together various stakeholders to evaluate and learn from an event and formulate process improvement.

Jim Crawley was a fifty-three-year-old man in good health who was finally brought into a hospital for a knee replacement because of repeated knee injuries during his professional football career. Jim had tried physical therapy, utilizing many anti-inflammatory medications and even a problematic trial of pain medications. The patient very much looked the part of an ex-athlete and still had the broad shoulders and wide neck that had helped him succeed on the football field.

Jim had resisted the idea of surgery, both because of the expense and the time required for rehabilitation. He had read up on Google about knee replacements and was discouraged. After discussions with his wife and two grown sons, he elected not to have the operative procedure and suffered for two more years, getting injections and taking medications. It was a stomach ulcer caused by the long-term use of nonsteroidal painkillers that exacerbated the issue and led him finally to the hospital for knee replacement.

Many older patients getting knee replacements are insured through government programs. They encourage outpatient surgery for efficiency of care but primarily to save a significant amount of money for hospitalization. Jim qualified for inpatient surgery because of his recent history of a bleeding ulcer that made him a higher risk.

As a gregarious ex-athlete, Jim spent most of his time in the preoperative area joking with the staff. They understood that this was, in part, his response to the stress of the situation but enjoyed his friendly and non-complaining ways. While in the hospital, he had an uneventful procedure (you thought it would be a case of wrong-site surgery). He was given a dose of Dilaudid in the recovery area for crescendo pain in his operated knee, which produced some immediate relief. After further observation, he was transferred to the surgical inpatient service.

After arrival at the medical-surgical unit, he was sleeping intermittently and required another dose of pain medication about four hours after his initial transfer to the ward. He got up with the physical therapist and walked fifty feet in the hospital hallways with the additional safety of a walker. On evening rounds, the nurse noted that his pulse was slightly elevated and that he appeared to be having some mild shortness of breath. Although she thought this might be due to some increasing discomfort he was complaining of, she called his surgeon, who ordered a portable chest X-ray as an initial screen for postoperative pneumonia or pulmonary embolism. While waiting for the mobile X-ray machine to come, the patient started complaining of an inability to catch his breath and chest pain. An RRT (Rapid Response Team) was called, and during the rapid evaluation, the patient worsened rapidly and proceeded to a cardiac arrest.

One of the intensivists and the emergency physician responded to the hospital-wide code blue call. In an intricate ballet of controlled chaos, the patient's nurse, respiratory therapist, and the code blue team performed cardiac resuscitation. During the thirty minutes that followed the attempts to revive Jim, the patient's orthopedist rushed into the room, having finished another surgical case. Seeing the respiratory therapist straddling the patient and doing chest compressions, he immediately called out orders. The intensivist snapped back at him that everything was being done according to protocol. The orthopedist replied, "But this is *my* patient," and the intensivist reluctantly retreated to the corner of the room, looking pale and chagrined. Despite considerable efforts, including CPR, intubation, and multiple rounds of drugs, Jim was pronounced dead, and the time was recorded. The orthopedist, understandably upset, started asking various team members how this event could have happened, looking for someone to blame.

An electrocardiogram just before his cardiac arrest showed evidence of what appeared to be a myocardial infarction (heart attack) in progress.

Jim's wife and son, who had just left for the evening, were emergently called back to the hospital. The notification of Jim's death was incredibly painful and was met by the wife's sobbing response and anger from his son. Neither could believe what happened and couldn't or wouldn't think there wasn't an accident or medical error.

Any unexpected death in the hospital is a tragedy for the patient, family, and staff. Risk management was notified, and the surgeon spoke immediately to the patient's wife, trying to console her, giving her the appropriate facts about why this could have happened, while himself trying to understand the cause of this unexpected event. An immediate investigation was initiated, and an RCA was called. The root cause analysis brought together members of all aspects of the TEAM that participated in this patient's care. The goal was not to assign blame but to better understand the potential issues that impacted Jim's care and, once isolated, correct or mitigate them.

Taking a patient to surgery is a highly complex affair. It requires multiple entities to collaborate before, during, and after the surgery. Medical clearance is needed, ideally coming from the patient's primary physician within the immediate period before the procedure. A certain amount of testing is required, such as an MRI, to meet standard criteria for surgery approval. The patient then must meet the standards of the anesthesiology department at the time of surgery to eliminate or at least anticipate, as much as possible, the risk of anesthetics and putting the patient to sleep. This process must occur within thirty days of the planned surgery to minimize the patient's risk of developing a complicating medical problem adjacent to the scheduled time.

The patient then checks into the hospital early on the morning of surgery, after using special soap during a shower or cleansing the night before and the morning of their procedure. This is done to minimize the risk of secondary infection from bacteria harbored on the skin. In addition, they have a mandatory educational program to prepare them for the operation and the postoperative recovery period and rehabilitation.

Theoretically, having an elective procedure in the hospital is safer than in a surgery center. This is why Jim, at higher risk, was operated on in the hospital. However, all procedures, whether in the hospital or outpatient, have some degree of risk. The risk is small, but having available resources to deal with an emergency immediately necessitates comprehensive risk evaluation before surgery to determine the relative safety of an inpatient vs. outpatient surgery center procedure.

During the RCA for Jim's death, the questions asked pertained to whether the care met the standards or opportunities that might have been anticipated or avoided during this terrible event. The key to the RCA was to get input from all members of the extensive team that participated in the preparation, delivery of surgery, and post-procedural recovery. Were there opportunities that might have impacted the outcome? Could there have been errors in his overall care, or was this preventable, were mistakes made, or was this an unexpected but unavoidable circumstance? This is all under the auspices of a Safety Work Product and is legally protected so that the individuals involved can bare their soles and openly and honestly discuss Jim's case.

In some cases, particularly in university or tertiary care facilities (autopsies are performed at local or regional hospitals on a much less regular basis), an autopsy, with family consent, might be performed to give a more definitive answer about the cause of death. This opportunity to have a pathologist examine the deceased anatomically, microscopically, and toxicologically provides the team and the family with in-depth information on the reasons for this unexpected and unfortunate outcome. Jim's family, in this case, consulted an attorney about the possibility of legal action.

In an HRO (high-reliability organization), every aspect of the care would be examined, looking for process, judgment, human, and system errors. Every part of the hospital and surgical care is reviewed, but prehospital care is also examined closely in today's medical world. In Jim's case, was the prehospital evaluation in-depth enough to alert the care team to underlying potential cardiac factors that compromised the surgery's everyday stress? Was the presurgical anesthesia work-up comprehensive enough to reveal cardiac risk factors?

Rather than looking for blame, which certainly is a gut-level reaction, the process of in-depth analysis can utilize a tool known as just culture. In some ways, this is counterintuitive, but it allows for a fair and just understanding of the circumstances of the case and potential appropriate action. Not pointing a finger, or taking punitive action, except in rare cases, creates a culture and atmosphere where staff is not hesitant to report errors, even when made by themselves. This is an opportunity to know from the best perspective the circumstances of the case, and in some instances, it allows for timely remediation that might be life-saving.

In his book *Zero Harm*, Craig Clapper describes a medication error case responsible for a young patient's death. "The hospital's response at the time of blaming employees instead of investigating possible systemic causes compounded the problem." Clapper describes just culture as nonpunitive and "one of shared accountability in which organizations bear responsibility for their systems and for treating team members fairly . . . and for team members to have the responsibility of speaking out" [(10) p. 143].

Mr. Clapper and his team have brought error reduction science to medicine, utilizing their experiences in nuclear energy and commercial and military aviation. They have focused hospitals on being high-reliability organizations. They present a tool kit to hospital staff of the "nut and bolts" of a highly effective functional program. HRO also supports individual staff growth in the principles of safety and its application in the complex and highly variable hospital world. Grading the severity of events and proscribing specific elements to an RCA has helped bring consistency and focused action to cases like Jim Crawley's.

During Jim Crawley's RCA, the team was asked to closely examine his care and look carefully for trends or themes that could lead to significant system changes in the entire elective surgical process. In general, this process represents a comprehensive review, followed by action plans to improve the care of all patients. The HRO (high-reliability organization) approach is not primarily a statistical one but is based on the belief that a serious complication is never OK, and the aim is zero harm (11).

In HRO organizations, we have worked a parallel process to the RCA called Candor. This consists of full disclosure to the patient and family by the treating team of events and circumstances that may lead to less than acceptable outcomes. One event can take center stage in this process and may represent the tiny tip of the health care iceberg.

One case can impact the entire health care system. One wrong dose of medication causing harm may change how the drug is given, where it is stored, labeled, and lead to safeguards such as checklists or double-checks performed before administration.

As we discuss cases where careful analysis and staff input allowed for an understanding of the errors and instilling improvement in the processes of care, the impact on the staff is also an essential focus of just culture. The effect on the team is also a core element of Candor. The death of patients often significantly impacts the hospital and staff. For certain circumstances, the hospital is the best place for a patient to die, and therefore it is not an uncommon event but is always accompanied by tremendous emotions as opposed to other industries where death or a less than ideal outcome is always an issue, these circumstances are a daily occurrence in the hospital setting. They do not necessarily, or even commonly, suggest error. This does not deter most hospitals from reviewing all such cases and looking for opportunities for improvement.

"As recently as 1945, most deaths occurred in the home. By the 1980s, just 17% did. Those who did die at home likely died too suddenly to make it to the hospital-say, from a massive heart attack, stroke, or violent injury-or were too isolated to get somewhere that could provide help. Across not just the United States but also the entire industrialized world, the experience of advanced aging and death has shifted to hospitals and nursing homes. [(12), Gawande, pg. 6]

The clinical staff is often besieged by some of their patients dying, and their acceptance of this ultimate event is often complex and heartbreaking. Gawande speaks about the medical education of physicians, but it applies to all clinical caregivers. "We paid our medical tuition to learn about the inner process of the body, the intricate mechanisms of its pathologies, and the vast trove of discoveries and technologies that have accumulated to stop them" (13). Gawande p. 3). The practice of medicine also demands our continuous dedication to death and dying in our patients, which only makes the emotional impact more real.

More and more patients are permitted to die at home because of the great work palliative care programs and hospice organizations provide. Dying with dignity with loved ones at the bedside is undoubtedly preferable to death in the hospital. Yet caregivers must deal with the expected hospital deaths daily and quickly redirect their emotions to the steady stream of waiting patients.

Most acute care hospitals utilize programs such as Candor to help focus on staff needs during such complex emotional times. The balance between ownership and detachment and accountability and responsibility among clinical caregivers should always be an essential aspect of the culture of a medical organization, therefore a focus of the first **WHAT**. The reaction of Jim's orthopedist illustrated in part his complex relationship with the patient. The surgeon had feelings of ownership and responsibility and had underlying concerns about his professional liability, reputation, and self-confidence. The first sentence in Gawande's book On Being Mortal is, "I learned about a lot of things in medical school, but mortality wasn't one of them" [(14) p. 1].

How we handle mortality helps us define our culture and **WHAT** we are about. Jim's death had to be closely looked at from safety and quality points of view, but it also needed to be an opportunity for staff understanding and support. Unlike other industries, with which medicine is often compared, death is part of everyday life, and its emotional toll is considerable.

III.

WHAT (AS AN ORGANI-ZATION, WHAT ARE WE ABOUT AND HOW DO WE FUNCTION)

Doris Lamore was a sixty-six-year-old female in the hospital for complicated foot surgery. When she was five, a car accident left her with some lower leg and foot abnormalities, seriously compromising her gait. A year after her husband died, she became increasingly aware of her disability, mainly how it made her appear. After consulting several specialists, she found one that felt he could significantly improve the visual and functional aspects of her standing and walking. She received authorization after several weeks from Medicare and scheduled her procedure. Doris dipped into her savings and purchased an entirely new outfit after much indecision in anticipation of her surgery. After years of downplaying her appearance, she chose a red dress that she would feel elegant in wearing once again.

Doris entered the hospital one early morning. She had followed all the preoperative guidelines, and although feeling anxious, she looked forward to seeing herself and being seen in her new red dress. In the operating room, she was given spinal anesthesia, but she received, by error, an injection of digitalis intrathecally (medication injected directly into the space covering the spinal canal). In most cases of a medication error, the patient can be observed without significant mishaps, other complications, or even delay of care. In some more severe cases, some antidotes may be administered to reverse the impact or effects of a medication given in error. In most cases, these lead to minimal symptomology and, perhaps at worst, prolonged observation. In Doris' case, unfortunately, the administered cocktail could not be reversed, and the patient went on to die. One does not want to see this more than once in a lifetime, if at all. These are the types of cases that an HRO culture addresses to ensure that they never happen again.

How could something like this happen? It should never occur, but hospitals in particular, and all medical facilities, are *dangerous* places. They deal every hour with complex and uncertain issues. Because of the wide variety of diseases, accidents, patient types, and the demand for fast and wide-ranging treatment scenarios, *the statistical probability is that errors will happen*. Safety has been termed a *temporary* moment when *harm* is low. It requires constant vigilance.

When my kids were very little, and my wife and I would watch them on the monkey bars in the park, I was waiting for a mishap as an emergency physician. There was little I could do but let them challenge gravity. I tried less than successfully to minimize my grunts of worry as my boys teetered between handholds. Complexity and uncertainty have been mitigated in the hospital through thoughtful and watchful and consistent behavior, checklists (Gawande), process redundancy, and alerts and alarms.

The conversation about safety and its evil twin action paralysis can be heard in constant discussion amongst the care team. The design possibility exists, partially within the EHR (electronic health record), with operational alarms and alerts and built-in checks and double-checks, to significantly reduce the chances of medical error. This structure has been very successful, for example, in the airline industry. It is a measured approach that includes pilot redundancy (co-pilot), frequently reinforced standardized expertise development, and rehearsed (simulator), which is consistently applied to the same airframe. This is backed up with instruments constantly calibrated, rechecked, and scheduled for mandatory maintenance. When combined with CRM (crew resource management), this translates into the beautiful recent airline safety record. We will talk more later about CRM. Still, it is a culture that encourages active input from every team member, even if they are expressing concerns not appreciated by the team leader. Seal team hierarchy exemplifies this shared action approach that is so successful in small highly functioning groups.

Safety in commercial aviation is an essential attribute but has a considerable cost, and urgency (being on time) plays an important but secondary role in the airline industry. The prices of the resources committed to safety are amortized and well spent when judged from a risk-ratio point of view.

There are some startling differences when air travel is compared to medical activity in the emergency department. Decisions are made under tremendous time pressure in both and can frequently be life-saving. Although on occasion, as a practicing emergency physician, I had the luxury of having a colleague or specialist "come look at this." Most of the time, I was independently making extremely rapid serious decisions utilizing a combination of algorithmic data, intuition, and emotional intelligence [(15) Coget].

Although the number of individuals at risk might seem to point at an airline disaster as more critical, the hundreds of thousands of unnecessary deaths in the medical field certainly up the ante. Those of us who have worked in the ED will tell you that, despite specific seasonal shifts, such as the predominance of the flu during the winter months, every day in the ED presents new, uncertain challenges with a changing set of complexity and variability. The airline industry has worked very hard to minimize the impact of these elements.

Paula Triffin was brought to the emergency department during a hectic day. Watching the nurses assist the paramedics in transferring Paula to a critical care bed in the emergency department allowed me a few seconds of thought. From the base station radio discussion, I knew that the paramedics had answered a 911 call to a residence. A base station is a telecom device that allows specially trained nurses to assist the paramedic evaluation and on-scene treatment with consultation from the emergency physician. In most cases, paramedics work from protocols covering many situations, and the base station contact is only informational. The paramedics reported, over the radio, that the patient, a thirty-two-year-old, had been found nearly unresponsive by her husband. Vital signs at home revealed a very rapid pulse of 130 and barely attainable blood pressure of 80 systolic. There was no evidence of bleeding or trauma. The paramedics immediately started an IV line for rapid infusion of fluids, put Paula on a gurney, and rapidly transferred her to the hospital.

Paula's transfer to an ED bed from the ambulance gurney allowed the time for a few seconds of thought. **Algorithmic data** that had become ingrained in my decisions, based on education, extensive reading, and published and taught benchmarks, were an essential part of my **Decision Vortex** (AKA the decision triangle). These elements were the cornerstones of my knowledge base but only part of my armamentarium. The second factor was, as described in *Blink*, **my intuition** (16). This skill, found in many experienced practitioners, was developed over time through pattern recognition that develops from treating many patients with diffuse diseases. The third element that came into play, as described by Goleman, was my **emotional intelligence** (17). I was fortunate enough to understand my inner feelings and experiences, enhance how I reacted and communicated with patients and their families, and help me understand how best to help them.

Dealing with Paula's distraught husband and his immediate question, "Will she be all right? I quickly palpated her abdomen and found it distended and very tender. "Could she be pregnant?" I asked. "It's possible," he replied. "We have been trying to have a baby."

The ED team was then instructed to treat Paula as a patient with a ruptured ectopic pregnancy, with emergent blood transfusions and a STAT trip to the OR with an OB/GYN surgeon. This was all done before receiving the results of any tests, not even a pregnancy test because a delay would have put the patient at incredible life-threatening risk.

The Decision Vortex is not infallible—utilizing algorithms to organize diagnostic and therapeutic regimens, combined with intuition and pattern recognition, assisted by emotional intelligence factors—but allows decisions to be weighed, particularly in urgent, chaotic situations, and allows for action. Following the steps of evaluating information as it becomes available, like blood tests and radiological studies, are necessary follow-ups to the initial process. In the ED, this is an essential skill set, but it transcends the walls of the emergency department and is helpful in all critical and time-sensitive decisions. Following protocols, standard practice, and even checklists should always leave room for the gut-level internal thinking of educated and motivated leaders, managers, and local staff.

Both emotional intelligence and intuition have some part in the decision cascade or matrix that we use in medicine to make rapid patient care decisions, often impacting life and death. It allows for quick decision-making. In some ways, it is all part of the heuristic model described by Kahneman and Tversky about decision-making in any field. Their model, which was developed for economics and which won them the Noble prize, also suggests that the more recent and vivid experiences would be disproportionately weighted in any judgment [(18) Lewis p. 190]. Recent adverse events, such as the unexpected death of a patient like Jim Crawley, would severely impact the future decisions of the orthopedic surgeon involved. However, there was probably very little statistical operational relevance in his death.

The decision triangle of a standardized algorithm, paired with emotional intelligence and intuition, is a theme throughout the coming page. It makes up an essential part of *organizational and leadership culture*. However, these three elements must be utilized by internal searching for any underlying *bias*, which may negatively impact everything from the highest-level executive decisions to bedside care. A *balance* amongst these elements is rarely perfect. The accountability for it lies in the cultural acceptance of the balance and the support of the individual staff in their efforts. They are going beyond the "cookbook" approach and *demand bravery, permission, and personal responsibility that define the culture of some organizations.*

Lilly Lucas was a twenty-three-year-old presenting with SOB (shortness of breath). Her father, a prominent staff physician, created quite a stir when he accompanied her at the emergency department. He insisted on the senior ED physician, and only this physician, see his daughter even though the ED physician was in the middle of an emergency procedure. The father would not let any of the other ED staff start the care of his daughter until first seeing the requested ED physician. The staff was not even permitted to place the patient onto a gurney. The ED head nurse interceded and, with much patience, convinced the father that the ED team would not initiate any therapy until seen by the senior ED doctor. Still, in the meantime, standard ED practice could be started. With her direction, the patient was put onto a gurney after she was undressed, vital signs were done, and an IV was placed in the left antecubital vein. This was part of a standardized process that allows rapid care initiation before an emergency provider's bedside evaluation.

In the ED, Lilly had a fever of 102.5, she was hypoxic (low oxygen), and, owing to her difficulty breathing and cough, she was initially thought to have pneumonia. Her general appearance was that of a sick young female. She had dark circles under her eyes and pale skin and was undernourished, inconsistent with her social situation.

The father's presence made a comprehensive physical exam difficult, and he refused to leave his daughter's bedside. What was possible without "embarrassing" (father's words) the patient by putting her in a gown revealed a heart murmur, which her doctor father described as long-standing. The ED physician had some difficulty getting a complete history from the patient because of her shortness of breath and because her father answered most of the medical questions. The patient denied drugs or alcohol, lived at home with her parents, didn't smoke, worked a regular job, and had no other real contributory medical history. She was started on antibiotics in the emergency department for presumed pneumonia and admitted.

On her second hospital day, Lilly's blood culture came back positive, and she subsequently had an echocardiogram that demonstrated a dysfunctional mitral valve with lesions consistent with bacterial vegetation. Without the father in attendance, more aggressive questioning of the patient revealed that she was shooting heroin. A more in-depth physical exam revealed evidence of IV drug abuse, primarily between her toes.

Unfortunately, Lilly's story doesn't end there. Lilly was initially admitted to the intensive care unit, where her deteriorating condition needed respiratory support with intubation and ventilator management. The first few days in the hospital were harrowing for her family, although Lilly didn't remember it because she was heavily sedated. The prognosis of the severe bacterial infection of her heart valves was very grave, and in part, it was only her young age that allowed her to survive.

After successfully treating her mitral valve infection with six weeks of intravenous antibiotics and treating her heroin withdrawal in the hospital, the patient was sent to drug rehab with the support of her parents. She was sent home from the drug rehab with the backing of her parents, drug counselors, and careful monitoring. Many of the services available to her came from the parent's ability to pay privately for specialized support.

After a few months of apparent success, the patient returned to the hospital with severe symptoms related again to a bacterial infection of the mitral heart valve (endocarditis). At this juncture, her valve was so damaged that she required open-heart surgery after a course of antibiotics. Unusual as it may seem for a young woman without birth or congenital defects to need open-heart surgery, the critical nature of her heart infection and the long, complicated post-surgery period demonstrated that her difficult journey was just beginning and that a positive outcome had a dim chance of success.

✦ Lilly's case was intriguing in many aspects, an indictment of our troubled times and an illustration of *bias*. Her social upbringing, her father, a doctor and colleague, and living at home in an upscale neighborhood biased the ED physician and initial treatment team. If a similar young patient were seen in the ED but was homeless and brought in from the streets by the paramedics, the role of drugs would have been a focal part of an initial evaluation. Did this impact the appropriateness of care and her prolonged course? Indeed, something to be considered.

Understanding my heuristic thoughts as an emergency physician allowed me to filter out my biases, or at least recognize and deal with them most of the time. Most of the discussions about *bias*, and the organizational imperative to eliminate it, are usually focused on skin color, heritage, language, body habitus, and sexual orientation. Eliminating this bias has become a top priority and is currently being recognized and resourced with some success. Patients that present with self-destructive behavior complicated by drugs and alcohol, as Lilly was, should also never be allowed to influence decisions about their emergency care.

Patients who present with obesity, a long smoking history, poorly controlled diabetes, or other behaviors that compromise their health have to be seen through an appropriate lens, allowing for accurate proper treatment and avoidance of mental pitfalls. These are some of the complicating conditions in our patients that we face every day. We train ourselves formally and informally to recognize them in ourselves and try not to allow them to influence our care. But Lilly's case illustrates a more complex matrix of potential bias based on our own experience, upbringing, and inherent cultural values.

Bias may affect all our decision-making. It can be quite relevant to bedside life and death decisions. It impacts how we look at our world, and it also impacts how we define quality and culture, and even more specifically the culture of safety. Bias affects not only our care of individual patients and how we interpret events but also statistical information and how we look at the avalanche of data that is now available. This is especially pertinent when we more aggressively start asking **WHY** (the fourth W).

The role of bias in the *decision vortex* becomes more complex when the concepts of Kahneman and Tversky are considered in understanding the limitations of emotional intelligence and, even more specifically, intuition. We have long credited our most experienced practitioners, nurses, and other care team members for bringing forward their intuition. A professional nurse or doctor can walk into a room, see a patient they have never seen before, and sense or understand their condition on the basis of multiple visual, auditory, and tactile skills. This ability is a tremendous advantage in accelerating the reaction to the patient's condition. However, Tversky and Kahneman (19), from multiple experiments, point out the role of inherent bias in decision making, initially in the field of economics but applicable to decisions in medicine as well.

Kahneman and Tversky also demonstrated the tremendous power of proximal events to impact our thoughts and feelings and, ultimately, how we make a decision.

When I was chief resident at a well-respected children's hospital on the West Coast, I was called to the executive board room to meet with the "family "of a very sick little girl with Reye's syndrome." The disease, thought to be triggered by aspirin in young children, had only recently been described. The patient was in our ICU and supported for severe hypoglycemia, toxic ammonia levels, and acidity in her bloodstream. I was predominantly involved in her care with the support of several academic pediatric specialists. Fortunately, she was improving, and her outlook was favorable.

The room was empty except for the hospital PR person when I arrived, which I found unusual and upsetting. The conference room door opened, and two huge gentlemen in suits entered. They said nothing but walked the room, looking around. Shortly after, another similarly clad individual entered, preceding a man with what I can only describe had an "Al Capone" hat pulled low over his eyes. He sat down, and I was beckoned to join him by what now indeed appeared as one of his bodyguards. He was introduced, leaving me speechless. I recognized him then from multiple pictures of him both in the news and in historical programs of gangsters and the mob from the forties and fifties. He looked at me from under the wide brim of his hat and spoke. "You are taking care of my niece, and I know she is really sick, but you have done an amazing job." I was still too stunned to speak.

He continued, never taking his eyes from my face. "If I can do anything for you, doctor—and I mean anything—do not hesitate to ask." With that last statement hanging in the air, he left the room, followed closely by his bodyguards.

As Kahneman and Tversky mentioned, this was a proximal event that impacted my bias and, therefore, my considerations and decision-making about my ICU patient with Reye's syndrome.

Claire Dorfson, a fifty-five-year-old woman, was admitted with extreme tiredness, weight loss, and complaints of worsening body aches. The care team worked her up with a significant differential diagnosis, including severe depression as the underlying cause. Dr. Blue, a consultant who was called in on Claire's case, immediately suggested Addison's disease before the report of her initial blood work of low blood sugar and the continuation of low blood pressure despite IV fluids. Her admitting doctors were surprised at Dr. Blue's diagnosis made even before testing and further evaluation.

Although quite uncommon, after some difficulty, Dr. Blue had diagnosed another patient with Addison's just a few weeks before. His clinical acumen was based on his great store of knowledge and academic approach but was also driven by the proximity of recent patterns in the former patient. In *Thinking Fast and Slow*, Kahneman refers to Herbert Simon, an early hero in the study of decision making, and what his take would have been on the physician's concern that his current patient also had Addison's disease. "The situation has provided a cue; this cue has given the expert access to information stored in memory, and the information provides the answer. Intuition is nothing more and nothing less than recognition" [(20) p. 237]. That pattern recognition is subject to time proximity to previous events, in this case, a patient with similar symptoms to one with a diagnosis of Addison's.

Gladwell (21) also points out that intuition is based on pattern recognition, but this might be oversimplified. It is imperative at the bedside for the practitioner to have experienced multiple patients with similar symptomology to apply his intuition. Medical school and residency go far beyond book learning and reading and understanding journal articles. The clinical experiences are the foundation of care plans, standardized approaches, and selected utilization of advanced laboratory and diagnostic testing.

Despite the academic inputs becoming the most significant elements of differentiation and categorization of a patient's illness, the opportunity to actually see multiple patients during the thousands of hours of medical education helps develop diagnostic intuition. The chance to interact on a human level provides the caregiver with a more limbic connection with the patient. This level of interaction provides a global sense of the patient, not just his disease, but his ability to react to it. The more chaotic, uncertain, uncontrolled, and variable the situation is, the more critical intrinsic, and intuitive understanding becomes.

Intuition can be extremely valuable, but the recognition of bias has spawned the development of multiple courses that caregivers must take to enhance bias awareness. As mentioned earlier, color, race, language, sexual orientation, and even obesity have become significant topics for staff education. This focus has significantly improved the medical community's awareness of these critical underlying issues. It took substantial self-awareness and continued education and support to position staff to utilize their experience and most recent inputs, use their intuition, understand their own feelings, and minimize personal bias. This is critical in decision-making at the bedside, but it also may play a significant role in data interpretation and focus, even at the executive level.

In some ways, bias at the macro level may impact even more than at the patient care level. Decisions based on operational or financial data may have much more broad-reaching consequences, where bias may play a covert role. We look at hundreds of data points daily, weekly, and monthly in the hospital world. The raw data comes from multiple sources, state and national data from the government, and multiple data rating agencies. In addition, we get data closer to home from hospital system offices. This data is then the fodder for process improvement and executive decisions about the operations of health care systems. What seems on the surface to be decisions made on the basis of data, the interpretation of that data may be significantly impacted by the biases of the individuals at the executive level.

Were the early considerations of diagnosis in Lilly's case of IV-drug-use-induced bacterial endocarditis impacted by the bias of the care team by the social situations in her case? Did her belonging to a middle-class white family and being brought to the hospital by her doctor father significantly affect the differential diagnosis that her symptomology suggested? These questions are impossible to answer, but hopefully, they stimulate our thinking about how much bias plays a role in our decision-making. Bias is an essential factor in all industries, particularly in significantly human-based ones, such as medicine, where ultimately it is people taking care of people. Kahneman undid the idea "that human judgment followed the precepts of statistical theory" [(22) p. 256]. "The understanding of any decision had to account not just for financial (or operational, or life and death) consequences but for emotional ones too" [(23) p. 261].

Kahneman and Amos Tversky introduced psychology into economic theory, but it screams parallels in medicine. Not only did they discuss bias in all types of decision-making, but they also weaved aspects of emotional intelligence into the decision vortex. A critical decision reflects the emotional connection of a caregiver and patient, which is essential in basic communication and requires a gut-level appreciation of the patient's emotional state and needs. It is also a reflection of the caregiver's emotional state. It might seem obvious that a decision maker is impacted by what happened at home before they came to work or an upsetting phone call they had just received. Most of us, but certainly not all, are trained to leave "baggage at home" and are aware of the potential impact of harbored thoughts and feelings. The upsetting phone call from home impacting performance is well recognized. Still, the prevailing culture of a caregiver's home or early events in their life may have much more impact on developing deep-seated bias.

The proximity of impactful events, as mentioned, to the process of decision-making also has a very significant role in the influence bias may have.

On a hectic shift in the ED, I was in the trauma room taking care of a gunshot wound victim. The patient, a twenty-eight-year-old male, had a significant ballistic injury to his upper leg. Although it would probably have devastating results, we were in the process of stabilizing his vital signs. Trauma room #1 was isolated by sliding doors from the remainder of the ED and was large enough for a great deal of equipment and the usual personnel involved in a major trauma event. In this case, there were sheriff's deputies in and out, monitoring the progress of our care. Focused on the patient's stabilization, I slowly became aware of the loud pulling of curtains and raised voices in the main ED. The deputy nearest the door peered through the window and informed us that multiple gang members had invaded the ED and looked around for the patient we were actively caring for.

"Shelter in place," he said, and we all crouched down or hid behind large pieces of equipment.

The sheriff raised his portable communicator and called for large-scale PD and the sheriff's emergency backup. It was only a few moments before we heard sirens, and the ED was filled with multiple police presence.

I continued resuscitation efforts on my trauma patient until he was taken to the operating room by the trauma surgeons. When I reentered the main ED, it was strangely quiet, and I was told to look into the attached parking area. There were nine gang members with their hands handcuffed behind them, lying face down on the floor.

The in-my-face activities of that day in the ED certainly had long- and short-term impacts on my biases. Being aware of my emotional reaction to that day's events allowed me to fulfill my commitments without hesitation to my patients and move forward into the future. Not recognizing my feelings would have had a significant negative impact on my care of patients. The sound of rapidly pulling curtains around beds for many years raised my concerns about my safety in seeing certain patients in the ED. Recognizing my emotions helped me understand which day's events affected me and triggered some tools that allowed me to handle the stress from the events moving into the future.

 ⸁   Danny Kahneman also demonstrated experimentally that, when people made decisions, they did not seek to maximize utility; they sought to minimize regret [(24) p. 261]. In economics and financial decisions, "although I would like to make money, I just don't want to lose money." This suggests that our interpretation of situations and data may be biased, but even selecting what data to look at may be biased.

The decision vortex, which consists of the triangle of algorithmic data, emotional intelligence, and intuition, when used in the medical field, can advance the accuracy of decisions, particularly in emergent situations that are often accompanied by chaos, uncertainty, variability, and complexity.

The previous discussion on the elements of the decision vortex was aimed primarily at decision-making by folks taking care of patients. The triangle's tip upward tip refers to standardized components and thinking based on historical statistical analysis and "benchmarking." The last is a "hot button" term that describes "proven elements" in the care plans: plug and play. The positives of this tip of the triangle are not forgetting little built-in alarms, elements of standardization for the entire team, and data that can be garnered with some ease and compared statistically with like situations.

Multiple studies, for example, on ED cardiac care, demonstrate the advantages of this approach. Data indicates that patients presenting to the emergency department with chest pain or other suggestive heart attack symptoms have better outcomes when evaluated quickly and subsequently treated emergently medically or with PCI (percutaneous cardiac intervention). An electrocardiogram must be done within ten minutes of a patient presenting to the ED to initiate the process. Based on these principles, the entire ED team is motivated to facilitate the rapid acquisition of this critical diagnostic test. This is part of *SOP (standard operating procedure)* and can be implemented with little thought or delay. The timing of the EKG can also be monitored easily and used as a measure of the quality of care. This is a rather simplistic but accurate description of how validated data is selected for study and how it can be used to impact, at least, the many processes of care.

Harry Lawrence was brought to the emergency department by his wife, over his strong objections, when he awoke at midnight complaining of pain in his throat and upper chest. At fifty-nine years of age, Harry was the father of three children, aged seven, nine, and thirteen. Their favorite family activity was long bike rides on the weekend when Harry wasn't overwhelmed by his work as a corporate comptroller. Harry was pleased about the rides since he could ride his specialized road bike that had been his excellent companion during many triathlete competitions before the kids were old enough to accompany him. "But I'm in great shape," he told his wife as she bundled him in the family SUV after he vehemently refused to call 911. Harry also reminded his wife that he had had a complete evaluation by his family physician to expand life insurance coverage only three months before. "I even had a perfectly normal EKG," he said.

When he walked through the door of the ED, the medical team was focused on patients from a multiple vehicular accident. Harry, nevertheless, was immediately brought back to an ED gurney, placed on monitors, an IV was started, and an EKG (electrocardiogram) was done almost simultaneously. After the nurse had accomplished a quick history of allergies and vital signs, the patient received a sublingual (under the tongue) nitroglycerine tablet. All of this was done before an evaluation by the ED physician, complying with standard orders based on recommended data sets. After the initial ED physician encounter, well-established tests led to a rapid move to the cardiac procedural suite (Cath lab), where an interventional catheter was threaded into his coronary arteries. Based on intra-vascular measurements and other studies, the diagnosis was validated as an acute MI (myocardial infarction) stemming from the blockage of his left anterior descending coronary artery. He received two heart stents to manage the obstruction. After being stabilized, he was transferred out of the Cath to the telemetry unit (monitored unit) for observation and continued medication.

All the steps in Harry's care followed recommendations from copious research and published experience. Every member of the team was well versed. Because of the complexity of care and the many team members involved, checklists were utilized to ensure nothing was forgotten, overlooked, or done out of order or inappropriately. Harry spent an uneventful night in the hospital being monitored, and the next day after discussions with the interventional cardiologist and the nutritionist, he was discharged. Things had happened so fast that the patient had no realization of how serious his cardiac issue had been. His challenge was to take all his newly prescribed medications, go to cardiac rehab, and understand that being in good shape did not protect him from genetics and lifestyle.

Harry received the highest level of quality of care, but he also achieved safe care. Unfortunately, as mentioned previously, in the United States, "avoidable failures are common and persistent" due to "the volume and complexity of what we know has exceeded our ability to deliver its benefits correctly, safely, or reliably" [(25) p. 13]. The previous quote was from Dr. Atul Gawande, who has managed to take the *checklist* out of rote documentation and introduce it effectively into popular literature and mainstream medicine. Also, from the introduction to his book *The Checklist Manifesto*, "that means we need a different strategy for overcoming failure, one that builds on the experience and takes advantage of knowledge." [(26) p. 13]Dr. Gawande's comments and Harry's story are extreme examples of the algorithmic approach, which consistently utilizes checklists, published data, and careful data auditing or collection to measure the efficacy of ongoing treatments and methods.

Harry did OK, by the way, and went home on medications to control his blood pressure and impact the "stickiness" of his platelets. He was asked to modify his diet (probably the most challenging task), given appointments for cardiac rehab, and instructed to continue to exercise regularly.

There are a few negatives to an SOP (standard operating procedure) approach to care, such as overuse of testing and an overreliance on pathways. The data from this approach, either process or outcome data, is comparable. It can be matched to a peer group within an organization, fragmented by diagnosis or risk adjustment, and then compared with national data. This will be discussed further in more detail but reflects one of the essential elements in data collection; we measure what we can easily collect. This is the same data that the government or third-party payers use to incentivize quality or financially punish those programs below the national average.

Intuition, the second point of the triangle, plays a significant role in the decision vortex, mainly when the time to make decisions is limited. Trying to define intuition is a challenge. The more experiences one has and the more opportunities to care for patients definitely improve one's intuition. It is the difference between "book learning" and laying hands on patients in the medical field.

There is considerable discussion in medical education about the number of hours a resident can work. There needs to be a balance between the number of encounters a resident may have and the number of hours they can work. Gone, fortunately, are the days when a resident would be expected to perform hundreds of hours a week to gain the most exposure to the highest number and variety of medical situations. This is a more organized and predictable exposure pattern for the newly minted doctors where they are not overtired and too busy to develop the other attributes of their skills.

Do the newly graduated physicians still develop the level of intuition of their doctor grandparents? This is certainly a question for members of the entire care team. An experienced nurse is worth her weight in gold (this is true even now with the overvalued gold prices). Similar words can be spoken about pharmacy, respiratory therapy, case management, radiology, different specialty technicians, and multiple other care providers. As a busy clinician, my patient care was enormously enhanced by members of the care team. There were very few patient encounters where I did not rely heavily on my staff's expertise and connection with the many faces coming through the ED. My job was to respect their clinical intuition based on multiple years of experience. It was also very much my job to convey to them frequently how vital their contribution was in the total care for people we had the privilege to serve.

✴ In most emergency departments, there is a specific job of *triage*. This common practice was derived from wartime situations and has undergone a modern update. A scene in the movie *Pearl Harbor* poignantly portrays overwhelmed nurses selecting and prioritizing casualties for immediate care. The other aspects of the scene depict the same nurses choosing some sailors so mortally wounded that they were given pain medication and shunted to the side. No matter how many times I have seen this scene, it brings me to tears because of the emotions it replays from my history. I had several harrowing experiences from multi-casualty events. Bus accidents and multi-alarm fires require a different approach. There is very little time for data collection or even systematic template-based evaluation. Time is critical, and intuition plays a significant part in dealing with these situations.

The triage person in the modern ED is someone with significant experience, who ideally has "seen it all" and has the intuition (pattern recognition) to be good at this function. The person's selection for this function is not as straightforward as it may seem. Many experienced nurses would rather be in situations where they can utilize their considerable skills in immediately treating patients. Some nurses may not relish the listening experience required to obtain crucial information. Many nurses feel much more comfortable, even in triage, with a systematic data collection approach. As Dr. Gawande has suggested, many would prefer a checklist to make sure that they miss nothing. There is certainly nothing wrong with these approaches, and it is probably the standard in most emergency departments, but exceptional triage nurses bring another dimension to the role.

In the third part of the decision triangle, emotional intelligence is also a critical component of the high-functioning triage nurse. Daniel Goleman, who recently has best defined emotional intelligence, has suggested that "empathy is social radar" and "at the highest levels, empathy is understanding the issues or concerns that lie behind another's feelings" [(27) p. 135]. This is the stuff that allows rapid two-way communication with a person who is usually significantly stressed coming into the emergency department. Empathy is one level of emotional intelligence and allows for *human connection* that facilitates getting to the heart of the problem. The patient arrives as a perfect stranger, with their internal fears and concerns, making a brief new encounter much more challenging to decode. Reading the spoken word and the modulation of voice, facial expressions, and body language is critical to deciphering the patient's cues that reflect their underlying needs. This may be so subtle that the patients don't fully comprehend their own messages. The key to the interpretation of these elements is emotional intelligence. Not to be overlooked is that EI allows the triage nurse to possess an intimate familiarity with their personal emotional terrain.

David Jones, a twenty-four-year-old, presented to the ED with a vague sickness, brought into the ED by his college roommates. As with most college students, David and his roommates had little time or interest in their health care needs. Their personal and medical history was unremarkable. David was still at the point in his academic life where he struggled to decide on a major. His original thoughts of a medical career were devastated when he received a D grade in biology. He and his "buddies" had been drinking heavily over the weekend, and as David started to vomit and looked peaked, they all joked about his big-time hangover. He called his parents since his roommates were not giving him much sympathy, and they insisted he seek medical care. Reluctantly, his college friends agreed to take him to the emergency department to get "IV fluids."

In most circumstances in a busy emergency department, David would be asked to wait for treatment because of his presenting symptoms and lack of risk factors. He would wait behind other seriously ill folks, particularly those at more obvious risk because of age and underlying conditions. The nurse might have classified him into a specific category, having treated hundreds of college boys with hangovers or even alcohol poisoning. Still, something about his presentation alerted her to something more serious. Rather than categorize him as just another stupid college boy, she was able to treat him with respect and relate to his presentation, even though it deviated from her personal moral and logical code.

David was brought immediately into the treatment area because the triage nurse engaged herself more fully and, at least on an intuitive level, understood his distress and response to it. In addition, taking more than just a cursory look at David, she noticed a few unusual spots on the skin of his wrists and ankles. These skin lesions suggested the possibility of severe infection to the screening nurse.

This triage nurse demonstrated a delicate balance between the knowledge about the significance of his physical findings, her experience and capabilities of pattern recognition, her emotional intelligence and the clinical and social factors in David's case. The triage nurse's *emotional intelligence* helped her balance the bias of having triaged two other college boys at a wild college party. As mentioned before, the proximity of remembered events is a powerful force in creating bias. This interplay during the stressful operation in triage makes it very difficult to train and keep a nurse with these skills. There is a considerable responsibility under very stressful circumstances and consequential staff burnout.

The registration clerk asked David some admitting questions, but because of the recognized possible risk of contagion by the triage nurse, the staff immediately donned appropriate gowns, masks, and gloves- PPE (personal protective equipment).

The emergency department evaluation included a lumbar puncture, and spinal fluid was sent to the lab for analysis. Blood cultures were drawn because of the high risk for infection, and antibiotics were immediately administered intravenously.

As it turned out, David, this young college student, without specific presenting symptoms besides fever and pallor and rash, actually had meningococcemia. This highly contagious, severe infection frequently seeds the spinal fluid and causes meningitis. Suppose David had been handled differently by the triage nurse in a very busy ER. In that case, this young man might have well died or have been left with severe disabilities from this very rapidly progressive and lethal disease.

In addition, there was a severe risk of his spreading this very contagious infection to many other patients waiting in the ED waiting room and to many other members of the emergency department staff. The few people who inadvertently spoke to David during registration were given a course of medications to reduce their exposure risk. The health department was also notified of the potential risk to students and staff at his college because of the highly contagious nature of his disease.

Well-published results illustrate that meningococcemia spreads like wildfire in situations like army barracks or college dorms. In David's case, no other person was seriously impacted, in many ways owing to the intuition and skills of the triage nurse and the rapid response of the emergency room staff.

There is a balance between intuition, pattern recognition, and *bias*. Classical bias is now routinely being addressed in most educational and medical settings. There are mandatory education sessions about race, color, age, and gender identification. Organizations are more frequently reaching out to individuals who can introduce distinctly different points of view and share them across a broad personnel field. These learnings do not replace longer-term family and social experiences, but they help bring focus and awareness toward deep-seated prejudicial and discriminatory feelings. This awareness helps tremendously in providing all patients with high-quality care and expertise.

We must recognize that our most recent medical experiences may also produce bias. David's case might have been decided differently if the presenting symptoms had been interpreted less effectively. In parallel, does our last patient, diagnosed with leukemia and its multiple presenting iterations, demand our focus on ruling that terrible disease in/out in every case? Does the last patient we have seen, a college student with a severe hangover, as David initially appeared to have, impact our judgment on each current patient?

The more critical the situation, the more urgent the patient's need, and the more intuition plays a significant role. As an emergency physician, intuition plays an important role, particularly in getting started in an evaluation, as with the young women presenting with an ectopic pregnancy. The need to start treatment on a patient was frequently literally minutes, and I did not have time to wait for confirming laboratory or even a comprehensive physical exam. It was undoubtedly my practice to "backfill" my thinking and increasingly rely on the analog elements of the decision-making triangle, as I had more time to dedicate to a patient. I am fortunate to say that, for the most part, cultural bias played almost no role in my intuitive strengths. In retrospect, however, I am not sure that those elements of my experience, based on the patients I had recently seen, did not bias me, as Kahneman suggests, particularly in the haste I needed to function.

The overwhelming number of patients seen in emergency departments are not true emergencies, not seriously ill, and not life or death situations. I did not want to miss anything, obviously because of the potential harm to patients, but also for the dread that I harbored. Should I have ignored my intuition and waited until I could follow the path outlined in the algorithm? Looking back over a long career, my intuition served me well by recognizing my bias and that I always looked for the worst possible explanation. I told patients I was a professional "worrywart" and mitigated my choices with as much information and insight as possible.

In contrast to the elements of care found in the algorithm, which can be subdivided into multiple process steps and measured possibly concurrently, and certainly retrospectively, the results of intuition are much more challenging to measure. As we delve into **WHAT** we know (the third **W**), we will be looking at process measures and start to understand the distinction between them and outcome measures. In evaluating medical decision-making in the variable, complex, uncertain world, the role of bias cannot be forgotten. More about this later, especially when we step away from the bedside and talk about the meaning of large volumes of medical data.

Emotional intelligence (EI) makes up the final angle of the decision vortex. EI was made famous in the 1990s by Daniel Goleman (28) but conceptually has been in the social psychology literature as well. In his more recent book *Working with Emotional Intelligence*, Goleman talks about the great divide between heart and mind or between cognition and emotion. "Cognitive competencies, which a computer can be programmed to execute as well as a person" [(29) p. 23]. This emotional component remains firmly outside algorithms and machine learning competence. He further describes the emotional competence framework. Goleman describes five areas: self-awareness, self-regulation, motivation, empathy, and social skills.

Self-awareness: Emotional awareness, accurate self-assessment, and self-confidence

- Self-regulation: Self-control, trustworthiness, conscientiousness, adaptability, innovation

- Motivation: Achievement, drive, commitment, initiative, optimism

- Empathy: Understanding others, developing others, service orientation, leveraging diversity, political awareness

- Social skills: Influence, communication, conflict management, leadership, change catalyst, building bonds, collaboration and cooperation, team capabilities

Goleman describes the skills necessary for organizations across the board but are particularly relevant in medicine. Here the end product is a human being with all their variability, complexity, uncertainty, and quirks, and the "tools of production or care" are also made from the same fabric.

Self-awareness must be the number one goal for caregivers at all levels. Individual culture, history, and *bias* cannot be eliminated but must be understood to cultivate a receptive platform to meet the needs of patients. Only then can genuine empathy be developed, and the operational skills necessary for effective communication, leadership, collaboration, and cooperation sustained.

As we progress through the following chapters related to the medical decision vortex, emotional awareness, internally and externally, which Goleman describes as "recognizing one's emotions and their effects, and "sensing other's feelings and perspectives" [(30) p. 26]. Part of this is recognizing one's own bias and the patient and family bias, as we pointed out in the discussion about Lilly's case.

The ability to *balance* and quickly utilize scientific knowledge, understand best practices, and follow established processes allowed the triage nurse in David's case to direct treatment and protect the ED staff immediately. She was also able to follow her intuition and her history of pattern recognition, to jump to the most worrisome diagnosis. Perhaps more subtle but as important was her *emotional intelligence*. She was self-aware enough to get beyond the potential bias toward a "spoiled drunk college student," of which in a college town she had seen plenty. She was not "turned off" by the tone and actions of David's classmates but was empathetic to the discomfiture of the patient and treated him in a caring and respectful manner. All these attributes combined to save David's life and, at the same time, protect her teammates.

The integration of the decision vortex and the balance of its factors is a critical component of direct patient care and is an essential building block of an organization's culture. In the chaotic space of the emergency department, the integration of algorithmic knowledge and process, intuition, and emotional intelligence is recognizable.

The decision vortex and its components should be recognized as an essential attribute of the culture, or the makeup, of the first of the five **Ws** in our cascade. This allows leadership the flexibility to allow for appropriate decision-making at the local level, not solely based on standards set organizationally.

As a clinician looking at my clinical world and my decisions in direct patient care, many were heavily dominated by the decision vortex and its elements of algorithmic data, intuition, and emotional intelligence.

Decisions at the bedside clinical level and extending through all the ranks of leadership are also subject to Decision Fatigue. Tobias Baer and Simon Schnall report in the May 2021 issues of The Royal Society of Science that "there is a tendency (in decision making) to revert to the 'default' option, namely whatever choice involves relatively little mental effort.... In health settings decision fatigue has been documented for doctor's prescription of unneeded antibiotics." (31) This is particularly true when time constraints are an integral factor in the decision-making process. This understanding of the vortex, with the added complexity of bias, fatigue has a broader variety of applications in all decision making and how we interview and select key personnel, how we look at process improvement, how we interpret data and utilize it moving from the third **W** to the fourth **W** in **What2Why2What2Why**.

How do we look at safety events and peer review cases and make them central to HRO (high-reliability organizations)? What is the best way to evaluate our quality and commit resources to do something about it, and last but not least, understand leaders' role and development?

We just interviewed a candidate for a vital directorship role in one of our hospital facilities. He had an impressive resume. The team interviewing him consisted of potential supervisors, executives, and peers. Because of the pandemic, interviewing these days includes Internet-based visual and verbal communication. It certainly beats a phone call but doesn't replace an in-person experience. During the interview, there was effective give and take, many specific talent questions were asked and answered, but we finally asked where he got his passion from. What followed was a brief but vivid description of some childhood scenes, which, from my point of view, said a considerable amount about the candidate. It allowed me to understand better how he would fit into a heavily team-focused organization whose ultimate goal was the care of every patient.

In some ways, the decision vortex is the first step in the process of management. It seems evident that decision-making leads immediately to definitive action in the emergency department. It is what saves lives. Recognizing that abdominal pain is not from indigestion or even from acute appendicitis but is coming from a dissecting aortic aneurysm leads to a choreographed emergency ballet. It is only with clarity from familiarity with an emergency department that one can make sense of the fervent action of multiple individuals from many different teams. Each individual has a specific role to play and is expected to take ownership and be accountable for their actions.

The elements of the decision vortex when internalized on a patient-by-patient basis do not translate as well or are as accepted when evaluating data or even management situations on a larger scale. This, unfortunately, usually inhibits moving immediately to action or even accountability on an executive or management level.

In understanding the role of the decision vortex and the integration of its elements, it should be recognized that the most challenging part is the conversion of the knowledge, the feelings, and the interpretations into action. Situations in the ED may differ situationally from executive or corporate leadership decisions, but internalizing the elements of the decision triangle allows for complete midbrain ownership and response to issues. The best understanding of a patient's condition or in-depth knowledge of the latest concurrent information or data is just a signpost toward a goal and the beginning of aggressive personal action.

ACTION

Multiple factors affect our ability to move to action. Some of these are inherent in the decision vortex and the competencies therein. In terms of emotional intelligence, we have focused on empathy or "an awareness of others' feelings, needs and concerns" [(32) p. 139]. This is paramount in understanding the needs of a patient in distress and developing effective communication during times of institutional stress.

The balance and inclusion of the decision vortex elements foster appropriate, timely clinical action in critical situations. The exact balance permits an active rather than a static culture that allows for a proper response to pandemics, labor upheaval, or changing social mores.

IV.

WHY (WHY ARE WE AS HERE AS INDIVIDUALS)

The patient and the care provider are both parts of the team necessary to act on the pressing medical issues presented by the patient. However, self-awareness, "knowing one's internal states, preferences, self-worth, and capabilities" (22. Pg.50), is the fundamental element of recognizing **WHY** we are here. This consciousness is also essential in the patient-care provider relationship regarding commitment, communication, accountability, and ownership.

Inherent caregiver *bias* is undoubtedly one aspect that impacts treatment preferences. But understanding emotional intelligence identifies a much broader context. It is about how we were brought up, the folks we interacted with and looked at every day, and who made up the "quilt" patterns we were familiar with. It also is about how we feel about ourselves. The role we are playing, our feedback, and our self-image. This has a major impact on our interpretation of our feelings about every individual patient. There is a huge conversation about specific "Black Lives Matter" issues. Although encompassing this issue, EI is much more subtle and impacts every patient. When it comes to taking action, these factors control to a large degree how we communicate with and treat our patients.

As a physician, I was spoiled by my ability to focus on the individual patient. I was, of course, as an emergency physician, usually pulled in multiple directions at the same time. However, no matter how complex, I knew my mission, understood my immediate goal, and felt totally accountable for the situation. I thought I had the tools to manage the patient and was responsible, at least at that moment, for the outcome. I understood the "triangle vortex." My training made me comfortable integrating my knowledge base, intuition, and understanding of myself and the patient.

There is an argument in the medical world that some of these basic tenets of care have been undermined by the current structure of care, complicated by the problematic integration of technology. This will be discussed throughout this book, and later I will be focusing on how to convert the focus on the patient into action, even more specifically, how to turn an activity into *outcomes.*

When a patient is lying on the gurney in front of you, writhing in pain from a dislocated shoulder, the demand for action is paramount. The short-term outcome is immediately apparent, and the feedback loop for the action taken stares back at you while you stand at the bedside. After administration of intravenous medication for pain relief and sedation followed by physical maneuvers, the patient almost always has immediate relief. It is often uncomfortable, frequently rewarding, but always dynamic. Fortunately, one does not have to leap through political, financial, regulatory, and organizational complexity to see the results of one's actions. This is the milieu where I spent most of my time as a clinician. It was very personal and intimate, and the outcomes were extensively tied to immediate actions.

The relationship I had with patients was intellectual, of course, but also one of commitment and, as mentioned previously, personal. It mattered greatly to me, the outcome of my interaction. This, in part, was what kept me awake after a long shift in the emergency department, thinking about my patients, often a particular one.

Arthur Black was a seventy-two-year-old recently retired physician who presented to the emergency department at 3:00 AM with a burning in his chest associated with burping. Per protocol, he had an immediate electro-cardiogram, as did all patients who presented with chest discomfort, but it looked normal. As a physician, he wanted to look at the tracing himself, and he concurred that it was well within the normal range. History revealed that he had episodic chest discomfort associated in his mind with certain foods, and other than age, he had no risk factors for cardiac disease. He was treated in the ED with oral antacids and had almost immediate relief from his symptoms. His initial laboratory work showed no evidence of cardiac damage and, by protocol, was to be observed in the ED and given a follow-up appointment with a cardiologist.

Arthur continued to be pain and discomfort free, and after about thirty minutes, he wanted to go home. He was quite sure that his discomfort was from eating smelts and was similar to his past symptoms. Despite my recommendation that he remain in the department for several hours and have a repeat EKG and blood work, he played the physician card and was released at his request.

Arthur had a reoccurrence of his symptoms at 8:00 AM and returned to the ED. He refused a repeat cardiac workup but demanded a gastrointestinal specialist, whom he had called personally, do an upper endoscopy to scope his esophagus. He had a cardiac arrest during the procedure, and despite vigorous CPR, he died. The patient had a postmortem autopsy with the agreement of his family, which was consistent with a massive heart attack.

My wakefulness while trying to sleep after an overnight ED shift was sometimes to second-guess my decision, but more often to think about the vicissitudes, complexities, and uncertainties of what I was doing. I was prepared intellectually and emotionally and embraced the care process. This was an essential part of the subsequent case review of complicated or very complex patients like Arthur. I cared; therefore, it was crucial. A majority, certainly not all of my peers, felt the same way, which has given rise to an ever-improving health care system.

Specific trends in medicine have undermined the personal and accountable connection between the care provider and the patient. These are the same forces that have also eroded the continuity of care. The first of these is the impact of the computer and the EHR (electronic health record). The positives of the EHR are legendary. There is no question that the possibility of sharing information between caregivers, hospitals, different health systems, private practices, and clinics is enormous. Having the ability to visualize an X-ray of a patient almost immediately upon completion, for example, no matter where the study was accomplished, brings knowledge and understanding forward at a tremendous rate. It also helps reduce redundancy and improve efficiency. Like the Internet, it has facilitated communication and knowledge transfer to the general public. I can see my patient's radiograph immediately, enabling my ability to act on the findings that I see. This example is repeated hundreds of times in our daily lives of patient care.

There are, however, not insignificant consequences. Many of these are highly technical and based on the attempt to enhance the safety of our patients, which unfortunately introduces time-consuming redundancy. In addition, psychological factors have resulted from this new relationship between patients and doctors owing to the introduction of the EHR and its demands directly in the middle of clinical care. It is human nature that the intermediacy of the computer has weakened the bond with the patient. It changes the focus. It competes with time and priorities. In addition to interfering with the very personal relationship between the caregiver and the patients, it diffuses the feeling of commitment and accountability.

The next and even more formidable issue is replacing the patient's physician with an entire team of care providers.

Hans Andersen, a seventy-three-year-old man, presented to "his doctor "with immediately worrisome symptoms, including vague neck and shoulder pain. After a rapid evaluation, the 911 system was activated by his doctor, and a paramedic and EMT (Emergency Medical Technician) ambulance arrived at the scene to take over the patient's care. After an initial in-field evaluation, Mr. Andersen was given an IV, a nitroglycerin tablet under his tongue and oxygen, and transported to the emergency department. An EKG (electrocardiogram) was electronically and digitally sent to the receiving emergency department during transport. In Han's case, but not always, the private doctor notified the ED physician and gave him a brief past medical history of the patient. In the emergency department, Hans was rapidly evaluated, and with the addition of emergency laboratory and additional diagnostics, he was admitted to the hospital. The initial EKG in the ED was suggestive of acute myocardial infarction (heart attack). A cardiologist on call was asked to consult on the patient in the ED, and after a brief evaluation, the need for cardiac catheterization was established.

The initial cardiologist called an interventional cardiologist who briefly met Hans Andersen, described the catheterization procedure and its risks and benefits and potential outcomes, tried to answer Han's questions, and then quickly returned to the interventional lab, and waited for further preparatory procedures. A catheter was placed through his radial artery in the lab, and the study of his coronary arteries revealed a significant blockage of his main artery supplying the heart. A stent was inserted to splint the area of blockage open, establishing near-normal blood flow to the affected areas. After completing the procedures, Hans briefly saw the interventionist for further evaluation and discussion, but then he was followed by another cardiologist and a hospitalist.

A hospitalist is a relatively new addition to the medical ranks. This specialty was born out of the need to have a physician well versed in critical situations and physically present to diagnose and treat patients in the hospital. A doctor in private practice might see relatively few hospitalized patients on a routine basis and therefore deal with diminishing skills to take care of such demanding situations. In addition, the office-based practitioner, faced with twenty or twenty-five patients with appointments on any single day, could ill afford to leave his office for an inefficient unscheduled visit to the hospital.

The hospitalist works shift work, and therefore the hospitalist assigned to Hans Andersen was replaced during the evening and night with another hospitalist, who is then replaced by a third hospitalist on the following day. The advantage of this program is a highly trained physician who is unencumbered with outside responsibilities remains within the hospital setting, immediately responsive to changes in patient status.

The good news is that Hans did well. The troublesome part of his care was that he was cared for by eight different doctors and a bevy of other care providers during his short inpatient stay in the hospital. The impact on the patient, their care, and their long-term outcome has been studied in many different settings.

For example, HCAPHS (The Hospital Consumer Assessment of Healthcare Providers and Systems), a post-discharge survey, evaluates patient satisfaction. The questions and the subsequent information gleaned cover a wide range of medical situations in the hospital. The questions and answers that delve into the patient-physician interaction, including communication, are often not at the most favorable level of responses compared to other aspects of the health care encounter. Hans gave a very high level of response grades to most parts of his experience; he loved the nurses and the bedside care he received from everyone, but when asked questions about the doctor, he was not so high, partly because he wasn't always sure who his doctor was.

After discharge from the hospital, Hans was asked to go to cardiac rehab, where his post-heart issues were monitored. He was guided through a program of physical exercise and activity that slowly adjusted him to "normal" life.

Hans is a success story and illustrates the psychological undermining of what we used to call the physician-patient relationship. Does this undermine trust, and does this impact the patient's long-term care? Or does it impact the feeling of ownership and accountability of the medical staff? Backfilling the prior caregiver-patient relationship with reams of paper instructions, access to Internet programs, and even patient-specific portals falls short of filling the gap.

In general, the EQ (emotional intelligence) score of most physicians, especially emergency physicians and clinical staff, is relatively high and is an essential attribute for patients' rapid and effective care. The same has to be said about *intuition*. Quickly recognizing patterns allows for a quick understanding of presenting signs and symptoms.

Direct patient care, the need to immediately translate thoughts into action, and the ability at the bedside to monitor results, make a diagnosis, and initiate immediate care certainly impacted Hans Andersen's outcome. Stephen Bungay often refers to the modern-day and historical military in his book <u>The Art of Action</u>. (33) As a student and author about warfare, Bungay had previously published <u>The Most Dangerous Enemy</u> and <u>Alamein</u>, he came away understanding that the battles he studied were basically between organizations. He developed a structure describing command and decision roles that mirror the organizational structure of modern health care.

As a clinician, I was both in command and control and management and staff for the most part. Once I had decided on the problem with a patient, implementing a course of action was rather simplistic. Although part of a team, I was the leader and could, as such, initiate a course of action. This action might be adjusted many times as the feedback of responses would be used to fine-tune, modify, or even alter the action elements.

The importance of a team needs to be emphasized not only during acute patient care but throughout the entire organizational structure. CRM (Crew Resource Management) is an essential functional element of a thriving hospital *culture*. Many stories illustrate this point, but a representative one involves Lorraine, a well-experienced nurse in the emergency department.

A brief emergency department evaluation of a patient and a review of the laboratory tests confirmed in my mind that further consideration of the care could be accomplished after discharging the patient from the ED. I told Lorraine, the patient's assigned nurse, to get him ready to go home. She looked at me and said, "You are discharging him?" Within a highly functional close-knit TEAM, this question is expected and not seen as doubting authority or judgment. After listening to Lorraine and the fact she had noticed the patient had an unstable gait when he walked to the bathroom, and a couple of other observations she was able to make, I admitted the patient for further evaluation. This was illustrative of bravery, communication, collaboration, mutual respect, the value of intuition, and the enormous scope of emotional intelligence. Utilizing all our tools and relationships, all types of communication, verbal and nonverbal, allowed us to stay afloat in the sea of pathology in which we found ourselves daily.

CRM is needed to function during clinical situations, but it is also necessary for complex administrative situations. An organization's reliance on only algorithms, standardized responses, formalized leadership hierarchy, and communication predominantly through technology limit the influence of intuition and emotional intelligence. These elements are permitted and even encouraged in a high-functioning corporate culture and leadership.

Unfortunately, the advances in communication technology further undermine the advantages of EI and intuition to some degree. If Lorraine had typed me a message in the computer-based electronic health record, I am not sure I would have reached the same conclusion about Hans Anderson. Still, I heard her tone, saw her body language, and could internalize some of her concerns. Her intuition had proven correct so many times in the past; that sense alone would have motivated a rethinking of my clinical decision. However, the direct gaze of her eyes and the intensity in her voice piqued my EQ.

In the *Economist* dated Feb 5, 2022 (34), Bartleby writes about his concerns about the loss of nonverbal communication in our modern world. "There are no good ways to compensate for these problems," he says, addressing ZOOM and other telecommunications. He describes several techniques to highlight one's feelings during non-in-person situations but does reflect on the subsequent decrease in the additive effect of emotional intelligence.

Andrew Locke, a fifty-seven-year-old man, presented to the emergency department during the 2021 Covid pandemic. Until just a few days before his ED visit, he had been going to work as a landscaper. According to him, he had a history of adult-onset diabetes, which was under reasonable control. He had been reluctant to access the ED because of the risk he felt existed of being exposed to the SARS virus in the hospital. He didn't have a cough but was experiencing muscle aches, headaches, and diarrhea. He had a slight temperature elevation on arrival, and his pulse and respiratory rate were somewhat elevated. The ED triage nurse briefly saw him, and a chest X-ray was ordered. He had a nasopharyngeal swab taken for a Covid test despite denying possible exposure. Despite feeling that the swab felt like a "brain biopsy," because of the depth the swab was placed through his nose, he was put in a room for further evaluation.

Andrew noted that the staff treating him all wore specialized masks, and he was also asked to wear one. He was seen by the ED doctor and further questioned about exposure. He was explicitly asked to describe his day during this interview, and the ED doctor meticulously questioned Andrew about the details. After multiple questions, the subject of lunch was brought up in more detail. "I eat on the job with the guys," he said. "Describe it to me," the doctor asked. Andrew thought for a minute and said, "We get our lunch from the food truck and eat together."

The workup revealed he was positive for Covid, and ultimately, he was sent to isolate at home. His case was reported to the health department, and they followed up to make sure he was appropriately quarantined.

Because of worsening shortness of breath, Andrew returned to the ED four days later, was reevaluated, and was admitted to the hospital by the same ED doctor he had initially seen. After nineteen hospital days, much of which were spent on a ventilator for respiratory failure, he received multiple medications and supportive measures, including kidney dialysis. As with many Covid cases, despite supportive care, Andrew ultimately died.

Andrew's case illustrates the uncertainty of what we do. This particular disease reveals an often-relentless journey to an ignominious end. The literature suggests a constant stream of readmitted Covid patients who were previously evaluated. Although trend data indeed suggest age and underlying conditions, such as diabetes, make patients more susceptible to the ravages of the pandemic virus, there are no absolutely predictable features as to who may abruptly decline following a period of stability.

Despite some miscues, Andrew was appropriately diagnosed and initially met the criteria for discharge from the ED. The decision to send him home was made with the appropriate information and careful evaluation. The ED doctor, in this case, had minimal tools in his armamentarium to take more definitive action. Still, it was not based on a lack of a defined path or reluctance to make informed decisions and implement care. While rushing around taking care of the crush of Covid and other patients in the ED, Andrew's doctor felt the feeling of dread that comes from personal involvement and accountability of Andrew's care.

One of the most challenging aspects of the pandemic is the terrible toll, short and long-term, it is taking on caregivers. *As discussed earlier, we own our patients, despite the fraying of the ties between the patient and the caregiver.* It might be possible to remain at arm's length when utilizing benchmarks and care plans. Still, it is impossible to avoid some level of connection because of the two other triangle points, *emotional intelligence* and *intuition*.

As a physician, I always felt accountable. I always felt very involved with my patients. We will get into this more methodically in the coming pages. Still, I ask you to keep in mind the role of accountability, taking things personally, and the commitment to take action on the more extensive palette of hospital operations.

Some of this has been diluted owing to our reliance on multiple team members for a given patient. The primary provider, the consultant, the proceduralist, the hospitalist, and the specialist all play a daily role in the modern health care structure. This confluence of health care providers, without a doubt, adds tremendous expertise to specific patient issues. The downside is the undermining of continuity of care. The assortment of doctors increases the risk of duplication, the breakdown of the contract between the provider and the patient, and the accountability and loss of personal focus.

Many artificial situations exist to prevent these detrimental aspects of this care pattern. Care coordinators, social workers, and home health care providers, just to name a few, have been introduced to guarantee some level of continuity of care. This, of course, then provides continuity that varies by situation and the availability of resources. The complexity of the patient issues also complicates it. The diagnosis, the patient's response to the underlying problem, the social determinants of health, and the availability of easily accessible communication tools can all be problematic in various patient care circumstances.

As a physician, my relationship with the patient had changed. My responsibility, accountability, my involvement all diminished somewhat. It was OK for me to pass a patient off to another provider, and unless the case was fascinating, I never really wondered what happened to them. Yet my internal culture insisted that I didn't stray too far from my training, my interdependence with my team, and my personal involvement in the patient's course. These elements helped me stay somewhat connected, and with that came a strong sense of *accountability.* At some level, this even became dread, that perhaps I did something wrong, maybe made the wrong judgment, that harm might come to my patient, or that I would be judged by my peers negatively.

In the face of complexity and even uncertainty, the feeling of accountability and the personal connection kept me highly motivated to do the absolute best for the patient. Many of the caregivers I have interacted with have reiterated these feelings. This too was part of the emotional intelligence that I, as a caregiver, brought to work every day.

As part of my EI, one of the many skills I brought to the hospital daily was listening. Far-reaching research has shown that the number one priority for patients during an encounter was that their physician or caregiver listened to them. Despite this knowledge, Goleman writes that "physicians need to sense the anxiety and discomfort of their patients to treat them effectively. Still, a study showed how rarely they listened. Once a patient started speaking, the first interruption by the physician occurred, on average, within eighteen seconds" [(35) p. 139].

The individual patient encounter is an excellent laboratory to demonstrate the elements of the decision vortex. Excellent patient care demands that benchmarks or algorithmic care patterns are integrated with intuition and also the sensitivities brought to bear by emotional intelligence. These are the elements, and the focus on patient care, that contribute to an efficacious culture in modern medicine. Despite the complexities, the dwindling of continuity, and the interruption of the contact between patient and caregiver, the culture of care still is apparent. For the most part, traditional medical culture can still be very personal and leads to effective action.

Focusing on hospital operations rather than individual patient care, the role of quality and safety, and the usual manner data is reported makes it much more difficult for the staff to feel accountability and personal involvement. The critical data seems disconnected from patient care partly because of the massive amount of information available from multiple sources in the current medical landscape.

The balance between EI, intuition and the algorithm corners of the decision vortex triangle is also critical in moving toward action on the larger stage of hospital performance improvement (PI). It is this melding of the "triangle" elements that addresses patient safety and promotes operational enhancements. It is also vital to understand command and control in the larger health care setting as well as in the one-to-one relationships between patients and caregivers.

The critical issues of turning information into direct action and subsequent outcomes, as with a patient responding to medications and getting well, parallel global decisions made at the executive leadership level. The connection between the information about a patient no matter what the balance of algorithmic data, emotional intelligence, or that derived through intuition is straightforward. The outcome is often immediate or well associated with the action taken. The feedback loop to the practitioner is also relatively rapid and usually quite obvious.

Leadership decisions often must pass through the labyrinth of corporate policies, standardization, politics, and human resource considerations. This often makes the desired outcome more complex and dampens the immediacy of action. Paraphrasing the lines from T. S. Eliot's poem, information is oft used in decision-making at the executive level rather than the knowledge potentially derived from it. Further, abstracting wisdom from that knowledge and creating appropriate direct local action has become more challenging as executive decisions are increasingly made at a distant corporate office.

CULTURE

Since our first days of medical training, the culture we have been inundated with is based on personal accountability, connection to our patients, and a heavy reliance on our ability to integrate the three aspects of the decision vortex triangle. Emotional connection, ownership, and accountability are also significant themes.

Many situations helped define the scope and culture that shaped my practice during my medical education. The days in the anatomy lab helped me better understand the fantastic human structure that I had chosen to defend. Starting with the dissection of the human arm, with the rest of the body remaining shrouded to protect my tender sensibilities, the mechanics of the human organism, its fragilities, and my relationship with it were better defined. The connection was very real, even when not in the lab, since I constantly smelled the formaldehyde of my dissections. So many experiences, like dealing with a dead body in the anatomy lab, shaped the culture of my medical world.

Early in my medical school training on a home medical rotation, I was called out to see a patient and family in a less-than-desirable neighborhood. My job as a medical student was not to individually take care of patients but practice my skills at diagnosing a problem and communicating with my assigned supervising attending physician. I was flying solo, so to speak, with my backup a phone call away, so I was somewhat uncomfortable with my prescribed duties. I parked my car and walked to the address in an unfamiliar neighborhood. I heard gunshots. I rounded the corner and found myself in the middle of gun-bearing members of two gangs confronting each other. I started to back away when they all noticed me, and with great trepidation, I stopped in my tracks. I was still dressed in my short white medical student doctor's jacket since I had rushed out of the on-call room when I heard one of the men shout out. "Don't shoot. It's the doc. Let him pass." That unexpected position of respect, even under those highly charged circumstances, has continued to be an inherent part of who I was then, in the middle of the night in South Boston, and today.

It was part of my developing an understanding of the unique role we, as health care providers, have and the accountability and responsibility that comes with it. Many such elements defined, over the years, the culture of care providers and the goals to which we aspire. It was an essential element of **WHY** I am here (the second **W**). It was a critical element of my internal culture, goals, and biases.

In the hospital or more extensive healthcare systems, the culture of care, and more specifically safety and quality, must embrace other elements in a thriving healthcare environment. The model of the practitioner taking care of the individual patient that we had been comfortable with is stretched when we look at the totality of health care. Much has changed from the formula of a single doctor taking complete care of his patients.

Hospitals, in response, have developed many processes that address the quality and safety of care. One of the most successful of these is the *daily huddle*. During this time, representatives of hospital leadership, managers of a given hospital ward, and key operators of a given service briefly discuss (standup meeting, so folks don't get comfortable sitting and relaxing) the immediate activities of the day, address hurdles and opportunities, and stress the culture of the hospital. Most of us have a definition of culture in our minds. Still, that definition parallels the famous Supreme Court jurist definition of pornography: "I can't really define pornography, but I know it when I see it."

Google has 3,710,000,000 results when looking up the definition of culture. The first explanation under the subgroup "way of life" is "the typical pattern of behavior of a person or group." This suggests that culture is not static, not just a description, but an active path within which we follow. In the ever-changing health care landscape, especially in the hospital, the reality of not being in total control reaffirms that culture is and must be seen in active terms.

If there was any doubt about what culture is like, reference our current pandemic. Chaos is abhorrent to the successful care of patients. Except for the emergency department, which in most situations is controlled chaos, hospital personnel and processes focus on stability and control. Covid-19 presented an overwhelming and out-of-control situation. Patients were dying in the hallways, and the staff was afraid of directly taking care of the sickest. This is not to say that the team's heroism was one of the few constants in hospital after hospital. But who would have anticipated that this heroism would become the centerpiece of our health care or hospital *culture*? This dynamic embodies how culture is not the tall letters and words emblazoned on the walls of our hallways but an adaptive structure that integrates multiple attributes.

Before the pandemic, I would attend multiple leadership and national hospital operational meetings. These gatherings were often held at airport hotels, so we could jet into the conferences and quickly return to our hospitals. Typical of airport hotels, not only did the rooms look exactly alike, but as you can imagine, so did the lobbies, hallways, and elevators. These locations were quite serviceable but not known for their warm hospitality. This was understandable since most guests were there for a concise business or travel-oriented stay. Exiting my room during my trip to the hotel conference center, I noticed, on the extremely long, minimally appointed hallway, several carts for the daily maid service. As I passed one of the open doorways to a room in the process of being cleaned and prepped for the next guests, the maid looked up, made direct eye contact with me, and wished me a good day. That little piece of direct human contact made the impersonal airport hotel facility into something a little homier, more welcoming.

A long story, but in one of my hospitals, culture is expressed in many ways. One of the mechanisms for this is that everyone on the staff, engineering, environmental services, nurses, doctors, technicians, and admitting workers take the time to make eye contact and say hello. On one of our TJC (The Joint Commission surveys, the chief surveyor came in a little early to get a flavor of the hospital. One of the environmental service staff, not knowing who the visitor was, approached them and asked if there was anything they could do to help, and then walked them to a conference room where the executive staff was waiting. After five rigorous inspection days, the surveyor gave us a glowing report but then stated that her first informal interaction with hospital personnel was surprisingly welcoming and open and characteristic of what she found at all hospital activity levels.

✱ What I hope is apparent in these two stories is that an organization's culture permeates all levels of manpower. It is essential in developing safe and high-quality patient care, but it also plays a considerable role in our employees, their health and engagement and what they feel. Shein defines culture as "observed behavioral regularities when people interact." He goes on to say that culture is made up of "articulated publicly announced principles and values that the group claims to be trying to achieve . . . and the broad policies and ideological principals . . . the implicit standards . . . and how the organization views itself" [(36) p. 4]. Apropos of the above stories, Shein also discusses the impact of culture on the employees and "how they perceive their relevant environment, how they think about it, and what makes them feel good or bad."

✓ Culture needs to be active and not passive, not just the elements described by Shein, the hallowed words and sayings on the walls, but be made up of limbic attachments of all levels of staff. What are the features that appeal to the *want* (**What** are we doing here?)? What is our motivation at a fundamental level? These elements can be visualized as a circle with a triangle in the middle.

✦ On the internal triangle are our algorithm at the top, emotional intelligence on the bottom left, and intuition on the bottom right. On the circle touching the triangle but separate from it are leadership, collaboration, coordination, personal accountability, connection, focus, and tools.

✦ The point is that these elements are intertwined, and any disruption undermines quality and safety in the care of patients. These are not only the essential elements of culture, but they are the signs that our basic midbrain is attracted to, the elements of why we *want* to be a part of the organization. It is the pride of ownership and a sense of belonging. It is the brotherhood of caregivers. At one time, it was only the focus of individuals at the top of the medical pyramid, but today's health care system includes all the folks running around in scrubs. Some hospitals and systems distinguish medical jobs by the color of the scrubs, and it does help identify the functions of different team members, but all of us function for a common goal.

✹   Recently at a community board meeting at one of my hospitals, the most moving and uplifting presentation was from the director of environmental services (still called housekeeping in less enlightened circles). He described the processes of room cleaning, sterility, and testing of surfaces for germs and cleanliness. Perhaps under ordinary circumstances, this would have been too mundane for members of a community board, who represent a wide variety of highly functional community members (doctors, lawyers, and Indian chiefs). But the pandemic has changed all of this. Cleaning, sterilizing, and the danger of exposure to the Covid-19 virus has focused the community on the importance of the environmental service worker as a medical team member.

The tools of the trade have changed, and the mechanisms to judge cleanliness have also been elevated. Infrared lamps and microscopic detection lights and new and varied cleaning solutions were highlighted. However, it was the human commitment and even danger that was brought to the forefront which earned a standing ovation from the board members. It was not the process improvement that so impressed our community leaders. The commitment and personal accountability of the staff were reflected in the EVS presentation.

✹   The recognition by the board of directors of the commitment and accountability of employees, even the housekeeping staff, highlights conversely one of the dangers that dehumanizing brings to medicine: the computer, in the representation of the EHR (Electronic Health Record), literally physically stands between the health care provider and the patient.

✹   Today, a physical doctor visit may be primarily represented by the back of a clinician's head while they document the patient-doctor communication on a computer. An exceptional doctor or provider may make eye contact for a brief second while utilizing the computer in front of them to document. Diagnostic testing provides tons of information but psychologically has undermined the physical examination and the actual touching of patients.

Telehealth patient visits have been a significant advancement. During the pandemic, telehealth has allowed a large swath of our community of patients the alternative for physically seeking care away from their homes. It has enabled disabled patients to avoid the situational demands that their physical and emotional restrictions have placed on their access to care. Watching such individuals in wheelchairs wait for the "little bus" to come and elevate them into the coach finally underscores these hardships.

During the pandemic, avoiding direct physical exposure to medical practitioners and their other patients probably eased the fears of many high-risk patients. Discussing patients in the hospital with their families and caregivers through telehealth platforms has perhaps reduced the exposure to unrecognized COVID-19. However, it has also skirted the physicians' in-person conversations and an opportunity to explain and educate face to face to the patient and family. It is often the family member who secondarily would be responsible for most aftercare.

Moving away from elements that touch people at this very base level insulates us from the feeling of accountability and connection. Of all the factors that make up our culture, accountability, personal connection, and ownership are the essential elements of *active culture*. If the public face of culture rests in the mission statement, then the active culture is based on how we feel about the organization and our daily work-life elements that matter to us.

Medical care is not, to use a basketball term, man to man. Particularly in the acute care hospital setting, each patient is confronted by a myriad of health care specialists in a uniquely choreographed ballet of action. It is the ultimate team sport and relies on constant *communication* and *collaboration*. It is the continuous passing of information, depending on team members, dealing with substitutions, and relying on new and different team members. A lack of continuity permeates not just the hospital but is apparent across the entire medical theater. Mix this in with the complexity of patient circumstances and illness patterns, the large number of actual "things" that happen to every patient every day, and the convergent multiplication of these factors earn the description of being statistically "dangerous."

Add to this the fact that despite efforts, the culture of safety in the medical world is weaker than when compared to other industries such as airlines and nuclear power. The pandemic has, in some ways, intensified the focus on safety in hospitals; the most apparent potential reason is the risk to the caregivers themselves, which starts to feel like a very personal risk to an airline crew or nuclear power plant operators.

Pre-COVID and Post COVID hand washing data from hospitals confirm the above supposition that personal safety rather than patient safety may be a more powerful driver. In our hospitals, hand washing was measured in two ways to measure compliance with safety culture. The first way was self-reporting, which was the most problematic. Our staff "felt that" they were washing their hands to a high level of reliability. The following mechanism for determining compliance with handwashing was direct observation. We were delighted with these results, which demonstrated over 90 percent compliance with hand washing before going into a patient room and again while exiting. In addition, the observed behavior before and after any procedure was also excellent.

To our chagrin, when we utilized a "secret shopper "approach with unannounced observation, the data was not nearly as good. Pre-Covid, despite education, process improvement, and even employee accountability, hand washing compliance not infrequently dipped to 60 percent. Even though this percentage reflects the national average experience, it is unsatisfactory. Covid puts the caregiver at tremendous risk, and this knowledge has vaulted hand washing compliance to 100 percent. Having a personal stake in the game has intensified our culture of safety. Perhaps this is a fortunate byproduct of our pandemic, but it is an uncomplimentary look at caregivers and the protection of health care workers in general. No matter how well-meaning we are, it is human nature that health care workers are currently highly motivated to protect themselves first during the pandemic.

A significant body of literature addresses our current safety environment, particularly in the hospital setting. This focus is expanding owing to the metamorphosis of medical care from a hospital-centric view into a system orientation that recognizes the need for health care education, healthy life-styles, appropriate screening examinations, and outpatient procedure and diagnostic centers. This is an addition to the safe and efficient, more traditional care patterns of in-hospital critical medical care intervention.

The major thrust for this change in patient care is not public demand but rather from the folks who pay for care, whether it is the state or federal government or private insurers. Don Berwick, MD was an administrator for The Center for Medicare and Medicaid Services. He wrote in 2011 in an introduction to a book *Transforming Health Care* about the Virginia Mason Hospital's progress toward the pursuit of the perfect patient experience. "Healthcare is hungry for something truly new, less a fad than a new way to be. We are staggering under the burden of too many defects, too much cost, and too much variation in care, all described with scientific rigor, and social commitment in the landmark Institute of Medicine reports To Err is Human (1999) and Crossing the Quality Chasm (2001)" (37).

The proper care at the right price has, as illustrated above, been the goal for a long time. During this time, the idea of safety, quality, and efficiency has attained star status for those working in health care. Increasingly the federal government, states, and insurers have devised multiple methodologies to encourage us to take better care of patients. Some of these programs, such as those through CMS, are competitive systems that compare data from thousands of hospitals in the United States and either incentivize or penalize providers for their work on the basis of myriad goals.

These programs have extensively been expanded over the years with a hospital-based focus. The apparent reason for the government's focus on in-patient hospital care is "Dillinger's law: go where the money is!" A significant portion of health care dollars are spent in hospitals, and therefore the "pot" is most resounding and makes the most sense to engage heavily. Over the last several years, private practices, clinics, and outpatient surgery centers have also been drawn into the payment incentives and penalty structure. The rationale for this is also financial; although there may be many good medical reasons for focusing on outpatient programs, care in an ambulatory setting is much less expensive.

Initially, a large segment of the public had significant resistance to significant procedures and minor surgery in an ambulatory setting. However, good case selection, upgrading of facilities, and the addition of well-trained staff have made this form of care safe and acceptable.

Good care everywhere is the ultimate goal, but currently, there are heavy financial reasons to meet the current demands for a safe, high-quality, and efficient system. How we get there is the fundamental question. Combining these three elements was known as the "Triple Aim", and much was published about them. In the early 2000s, this was a relatively new concept and gained notoriety, particularly relative to published data about hundreds of thousands of unnecessary hospital deaths. Since then, there has been an addition of patient and caregiver satisfaction as an additional factor to the three previously mentioned, named "The Quadruple Aim" (Institute for Healthcare Improvement).

- Improving population health: preventing and managing prevalent, costly, and chronic diseases.

- Enhancing patient experience: motivating and engaging patients to play an active role in their care to improve outcomes and safety.

- Reducing cost of care: reducing resource utilization and readmissions while assuming more significant risk.

- Improving provider satisfaction: providing access to tools and resources to address provider burden and burnout.

The elements overlap, and implementing one aspect of the quadruple aim impacts the other components. However, the approach to each is slightly different in scope and even in data collection and analysis. Yet, much in the same way that the culture impacts individual patient care, so does the quadruple aim.

In the approach to patient safety, high-quality efficient care, and patient satisfaction, our success depends on our culture, in each department, on each campus, within each health care system, and nationally. In addition, understanding our ultimate goal, why we all come to work, and how we measure our success are key elements in staff satisfaction.

WHAT2WHY2WHAT2WHY2WHAT is a device to make sure all our priorities are in line. The first two elements we discussed reflect what we are doing here and **WHY** we are here. This **WHY**, as reflected in the quadruple aim of provider satisfaction, strengthens the resolve to understand the midbrain connection of our staff and the impact of emotional intelligence, intuition, and bias. If these elements are not clearly defined and articulated, the entire **W** cascade will not come to fruition.

What is our overarching goal? It is not enough to shout this from the rooftops or repeat it at every opportunity, but it must be demonstrated and believable. It is not enough to be in the mission statement repeated at meetings. But it must be consistent and honest to even the "lowest" team member. The goal must be simple, straightforward, and obvious. This is particularly difficult in the hospital environment owing to its complexity, statistical uncertainties, and multiple stakeholders. Success is based on leadership, communication, and the development of an executive and management team fully invested in **WHAT** we are doing here. How is it defined, and how is it articulated? This approach firmly puts leadership and culture in the crosshairs. The culture of the organization establishes the goal, and it is the leadership that defines how we get there. Leadership is not limited to the CMO (chief medical officer) or the executive team. Still, it is represented by multiple layers of leaders, many of whom do not even have director or manager titles.

Is the leader firmly vested in the goal? One of the hospital organizations I was part of had a very articulate and outspoken leader. He talked about patient care but spent most of the time in endless meetings about grades and financial impact. Being told that quality would be focused on in the last thirty minutes of a two-hour session and then only getting fewer than five minutes to articulate a few highlights and issues was a booming and clear message.

✴ Whatever was verbal or in document form about quality issues paled next to the leadership prioritization of the other more important subjects. "The most powerful mechanisms that founders, leaders, managers, and parents have available for communicating what they believe in or care about is what they systematically pay attention to" [(38) Schein p. 184]. In the highly competitive world of business and the highly intense world of health care, it is the formula: effort × time = outcome.

As we move toward a more in-depth conversation about the five **Ws** (**What2Why2What2Why2What**), we cannot underestimate the importance of understanding our goal. It answers what we are doing here (our first **W**). It is a recognition of our vision. The mission comes later as we define this more ✴ in terms of process. In his book <u>Start with Why</u>, Simon Sinek helps explain the difference between mission and vision: "The vision is the public statement of the founder's intent. Why the company exists is the vision of a future that does not yet exist. The mission statement describes the route, the guiding principles-How the company intends to create that future" [(39) Sinek p. 142]. Although there is much written and spoken about culture, it stems directly from the goal of the organization. It must be elucidated and supported by appropriate focus and resources. This is the purview of leadership. It can be split or shared, but it is the most critical element in delivering the **WHAT**.

Perhaps a more explicit way of thinking about culture and the current times we face is the concept of an active rather than passive (static) culture. ✴ This is defined in part by our goals. The pandemic has forced us to broaden and recast our goals by refocusing those most important to us. Staff safety, which has always been a concern before the pandemic, has become one of our core values. We watch staff heroically perform at the bedside of our sickest and most contagious patients. It is not enough to provide appropriate PPE (personal protective equipment) and demand adherence to policy but to understand the potential risk for staff and their families and the need for significant psychological and work-life balance support.

✴ In addition, our focus previously was predominately one patient at a time: the best experience, the best care, and the most current technology and methodology. The pandemic has caused a refocus to include the health and safety of the entire community. Re-tasking physical resources, finding unique ways to enhance isolation, surveillance, and finally, the large-scale vaccination of personnel has been an amazing challenge. This has been accomplished internally and in parking lot clinics, drive-through immunization centers, and enhanced telemedicine capabilities. These and other elements all reflect operational changes but with the maintenance of inherent cultural mores.

With the tremendous attention on outcomes and the "grades" that health care systems and hospitals receive from a myriad of governmental and non-governmental agencies, it is easy to get lost in the process of care and the scorecards as our ultimate goal. Our goal must always be purpose-driven.

Both purpose and process are tremendously challenging to control. We commit our efforts to this because the process is more functionally elegant and much easier to measure. As we have illustrated at the bedside, this is true and quite functional, but the process on the larger stage of quality and safety tends to divert us from our overall goal.

We must look to our culture to ensure that we do not lose sight of our purpose, and much of that depends on leadership. Leaders not only have to demand the discussion and definition of our goal but implement a system that carries it further into action. "The ability to motivate people is not, in itself, difficult. It is usually tied to some external factor. Tempting incentives or threats of punishment will often elicit the behavior we desire," Simon Sinek says, "but great leaders, in contrast, can inspire people to act" [(40) p. 6].

The presence of a great leader does not necessarily guarantee a vital culture, but the association is very well documented in multiple industries. It may not seem that way when looking at bedside care or the medical industry. Still, despite the uncertainties and complexities of health care, the leader is directly in the vortex of institutional success and is essential in delivering safe and high-quality care for every patient every day.

Kouzes and Posner, in their classic book The Leadership Challenge, define at great length the five practices and ten commitments of leadership [(41) p.

22]. Although the purpose of this book is not to rehash the well-defined qualities of a good leader, it is essential to realize that the milieu for a culture of quality and safety, at every level, starts with the leader. Briefly, as described by Posner, the five elements of practice are "Model the Way," "Inspire a Shared Vision," "Challenge the Process," "Enable Others to Act," and "Encourage the Heart."

The ten commandments (commitments) as per Kouzes and Posner are as follows:

- Find your voice by clarifying your values.

- Set an example by aligning actions with shared values.

- Envision the future by imagining exciting and ennobling possibilities.

- Enlist others in a common vision by appealing to shared aspirations.

- Search for opportunities by seeking innovative ways to change, grow, and improve.

- Experiment and take risks by constantly generating small wins and learning from mistakes.

- Foster collaboration by promoting goals and building trust.

- Strengthen others by sharing power and discretion.

- Recognize contributions by showing appreciation for individual excellence.

- Celebrate the values and victories by creating a spirit of community.

The leadership challenge is a very personal one and is meant to internalize elements that are very dependent on midbrain connections. The response to these fundamentals is then mirrored by other organizational leaders and members of larger teams. It is not only an inspiration for action, but also for emotions. These emotions become the heart of accountability, commitment, and ownership.

Leadership may also be characterized more traditionally by whether it is *transactional* or *transformational*, or, as is usually the case, a changing balance between both characteristics. This description is more about style than about leadership heart. Understanding an organization and its leadership structure may be more difficult as the size and distance from individual hospitals increase, as we now see in large multistate healthcare systems.

- Transactional leaders
    - Action-oriented
    - Contingent reward and punishment system
    - Accepts current structure
    - Management by exception
    - Tends toward inflexibility
    - Supervises and gives precise directions
    - Fits nicely in a hierarchal format
    - Rewards are usually financial or promotional
- Transformational leaders
    - Inspires through charisma and enthusiasm
    - Pays attention to the developmental needs of individuals and staff
    - Place a high value on creativity
    - Vision and goals are valued more than the bottom line
    - Embrace trust and empowerment

Transactional leadership attributes tend to do well in a health care environment because of the need for stability, consistency, and a finite, almost calculated reward system. As independent hospitals have been actively drawn into increasingly large and geographically distributed health care systems, the focus has been on transactional leadership. Transactional leaders feel very comfortable working within a standardized corporate approach and are rewarded for unanimity.

Transformational leadership has become less valued, particularly outside the C-suite, or noncorporate executive ranks. This continues to be the trend with the pressure to meet large-scale corporate goals. Unfortunately, the very nature of transactional leadership tends to undermine the recognized value of emotional intelligence, intuition, and bravery.

Transactional leadership is more typical of *static culture*, while transformational leadership is the centerpiece of *active culture*.

I spent many years in an organization with a mighty leader. His great strength was in challenging the process. And he constantly "searched for opportunities by seeking innovative ways to change, grow and improve" [(42) p. 22], yet working for him brought back images of my watching the Macy's Thanksgiving Day parade as a kid. The bands, the floats, the horses, and even elephants paraded down 5th avenue in New York City. With great fanfare, the parade passed slowly for what seemed like hours. At the end, of course unheralded, were scores of sanitation workers pushing huge garbage cans on wheels and utilizing push brooms and shovels to pick up the refuse, including horse and elephant droppings.

The parade's focus was the mesmerizing drama, the variety, the sounds, and the energy, but what was lost was the attention to detail of every participant and, more importantly, the lasting effects of the visible elements. This particular leader's nature did not permit an environment of trust and empowerment. His vision needed to be a product of significant input and deliberation. His leadership style was one of intimidation and a financially rewarded focus. As with the parade, considerable time and resources were spent "cleaning up the mess" after decisions were made without a complete understanding or even interest in their unexpected outcomes.

⁎ This leader was a perfect example of a transactional leader. His short-term impact, often very dramatic, did not engender loyalty, enthusiasm, or creativity. Perhaps these elements were previously not highly touted in a medical environment, but the pandemic has taught us the absolute need for them. Without the staff's commitment, under the most challenging and demanding circumstances, many more patients would have died and would not have been able to receive care. This does not occur without a deep midbrain connection. It does not happen because of dollars, sentiment, or union negotiations, but commitment, connection, trust, and human feelings.

✳ Perhaps leadership in the medical setting depends even more on *trust* than anything else if viewed as a two-way street. It is essential that patients feel a deep sense of confidence for those, directly and indirectly, caring for them. Trust is also a core factor for staff at all levels in that they can trust their ability to express their needs, perceptions, and even feelings in the pursuit of excellence in their jobs. Ultimately trust in leadership, not just operationally but at an emotional level, is key to organizational success. According to Simon Sinek, "Historically, trust has played a bigger role in advancing companies and societies than skill set alone" [(43) Sinek p. 104]. The environment of mutual trust is also essential. Leadership must trust, executives must trust, management must trust, and so on.

I regularly participated in monthly regional meetings. Approximately twenty-five executives and directors attended these gatherings representing the operations of hospitals and outpatient practices and facilities such as surgery centers. Most of us spent considerable time preparing reports from the various operations and systems for which we were responsible. Usually, we got a heavy dose of whatever the regional president had on his mind, so much of the session was spent listening and even taking a few notes.

On one occasion, one of the operational leaders did not have the "right answers" for some issues that occurred under his purview. The president spent an excessive amount of time "roasting the senior vice president," so much so that the operational leader passed out. In attendance, most of us didn't realize his plight until he fell out of his chair and hit the floor. At the meeting, in their administrative roles, several physicians rushed to his aide. My contribution was barking orders from across the room since the other physicians had already evaluated the situation. Fortunately, after a brief visit to the emergency department, no other evidence of pathology was found except for psychic trauma. The leader took a quick pause and continued the meeting without further interruption.

I mention this incident because it exemplified the toxic element of his leadership. A fantastic leader in some respects, but his weaknesses in his transformational and emotional intelligence undermined his effectiveness and the functionality of the entire leadership team. The long-term impact, not only to the unfortunate recipient of the president's tirade but to all the leadership that witnessed it, has been substantial.

Following these events, a president of one of our hospitals complained explicitly that the divisional leader did not trust her either. Consequently, that undermined her psychological ability to make rapid and brave decisions.

In the previously described circumstances, the powerful leader's style permeated the entire institution and impacted even at the patient bedside and upward throughout the organization. Most importantly, it undermined or diminished accountability and the personal commitment from those operationally tasked and responsible for the well-being of patients.

In his influential book on leadership, Michael Frisina discusses elements of the leadership model that rely heavily on the leader's emotional intelligence and suggests that "self-awareness is the first principle of influential leadership." The brain again is called to task because the ability to look at oneself truthfully and perhaps even change our behavior is challenging. "Once the brain learns consistent patterns of behavior, even dysfunctional ones, it hangs on to those patterns which are phenomenally strong" [(44) p. 24]. Listening to others, taking input, and, more importantly, understanding oneself are critical to leadership. Unfortunately, "talk to the hand" became a mantra with this leader, and his style far outdistanced even his most ingrained biases.

Both the initial **WHAT** and the **WHY** of the **W** cascade become muddled if the intuitional culture, the mission, and the vision reflected by the leader are not portrayed. "Influential leaders are keenly aware of the need to create an organizational culture in which people are encouraged to take personal responsibility for doing their jobs well and be accountable for their actions" [(45) p. 27]. This last statement takes us deeper into the **W** cascade of making things happen. Clearly, it outlines the role of leadership and what we are doing in the organization that promotes personal loyalty, commitment, action, and passion.

Danna Stewart RN, DNP, was the associate director of nursing at one of my hospitals. She was relatively new to the hospital, having arrived only several months before from a teaching hospital in a large metropolitan area. She was academic and highly organized in her approach and had started to make real improvements in the nursing units under her leadership. Danna had come from a historically successful, educated, and even published family and brought her energy to work daily.

Her staff, however, was struggling with her and found her to be dogmatic and authoritarian, to the point that a petition of complaint was signed by most of the nurses under her command. Many of her nurses had been in their positions for a long time and had enjoyed a "family style" atmosphere at work. Fortunately, "life hit," and the third wave of Covid-19 hit the hospital hard. Danna changed from wearing her well-styled outfits and began wearing scrubs. She was on the floors most days and even into the nights helping at every level, bedpans included.

Danna made this change because of the demands of the pandemic more than she did because she had the emotional intelligence to understand her leadership challenge. The proximity, her participation as one of the working clinical staff, the forced communication, and the identification with the other nurses started a chain of events that she was intelligent enough to take advantage of. The chaos and demands of Covid placed everyone, including Danna, in a position of mutual dependency and altered the terrain sufficient to reach everyone at a midbrain level. Empathy, respect, caring, and greater self-awareness during Covid precipitated Danna and her team's new pathways.

Danna's style was very transactional. This is most typical of managers, where getting through the day is the goal most functionally and efficiently.

This deviates from the definition of outstanding leadership, where a more extended vision helps to energize the staff. The empathy found with developed emotional intelligence helps communicate, in human business-like medicine, the language of relationships with peers and patients. These are the midbrain building blocks of highly functioning teams.

4. Good leaders are not necessarily good managers, and balance is the key to maintaining an active culture. Responding to uncertainty and deviation, from a global perspective, without losing sight of short-term goals, and commanding a vision without the loss of empathy, trust, and connection is the ultimate test of leadership.

Leadership and its challenges are seen in the C-suite and, as with Danna, daily throughout an organization. Reflecting on the decision vortex triangle and the surrounding circle, the leadership qualities embodied therein can be further elucidated. The first is knowledge and data-driven. The constant discussion when choosing a new leader, for example, a chief executive officer, is about background, experience, education, and other attributes usually articulated in great detail on the curriculum vitae or resume. This is often checked with references and an in-depth understanding and evaluation of a body of previous work. It is a pretty good guide for choosing a leader, mainly when an experienced interview panel is utilized in the selection process.

Related to a candidate's experience is their *intuition*, another corner of the triangle. This, as described in <u>Blink,</u> (46) is somewhat complex but boils down to pattern recognition. Clinical experience, crossing barriers, successful past problem solving, and even failures prepare an individual to use their "gut" to help make difficult or rapid decisions when data and algorithmic decision-making are either not available or confusing.

The potential trap for using one's intuition is the *bias* that we all potentially bring to any situation, choice, or decision. Overreacting to one's intuition, and the impact of an immediate environment and circumstances must be balanced by the experience that is reflected as intuition. David Myers raises warning signs in his text <u>Exploring Social Psychology</u> and reflects on "mental processes that are put into motion by features of the environment and that operate outside of conscious awareness and guidance." [(47) Pg 71]

The remaining corner of the triangle, as described earlier, is emotional intelligence. It is an essential element in medical decision-making, but it is also pivotal in leadership as a base for *active* rather than *passive* (static) culture. Goleman and his co-authors in <u>Primal Leadership</u> outline leadership elements that define an active culture.

- Self-awareness

- Self-management

- Social awareness

- Relationship management

"These EI competencies are not innate talents, but learned abilities, each of which has a unique contribution to making leaders more resonant, and therefore more effective" [(48) p. 38].

Goleman goes on to describe the capabilities within each of these categories. Self-awareness is the key element of the leadership model and of the first **WHAT** in our **W** cascade. Still, it also is an essential element of **WHY**, the second **W**, as individuals, we choose to function in a medical/hospital environment. From a leadership perspective and for the rest of us, what drives us are very midbrain functions. How we feel about what we do helps us gravitate to a particular culture, a specific leadership style, and therefore understanding our emotional intelligence to find our proper place and be successful in our efforts.

Goleman describes the neurophysiology that is the basis of our feelings.

"The thinking brain evolved from the limbic brain and continues to take orders from it when we perceive a threat or under stress. The trigger point for these compelling emotions is the amygdala, a limbic brain structure that scans what happens to us moment to moment, ever on the alert for emergencies. As our radar for emotional emergencies, the amygdala can command other parts of the brain, including rational centers in the neocortex, for immediate action if it perceives a threat" [(49) Primal Leadership p. 28].

This suggests a base of emotional responses that drive our decisions and culture. There are then two elements of this that are concerning. The first from Goleman, and then further elucidated by the work of Kahneman and Tversky, is that genetically our midbrain tends to function from a fearful or negative space. The Fight- or- flight response trumps all other feelings. The research illustrates how PET scans or MRIs light up anatomically place the amygdala in the middle of this conversation. Kahneman and Tversky, in a nonmedical setting, describe decision-making as heavily influenced by the negative or by "worst-case scenario" thinking. Choosing investments, their research demonstrated, seems to be heavily influenced by trying not to make a wrong decision rather than making a favorable or good decision.

Not making a wrong decision has extra consequences when dealing with direct patient issues. The reality is that clinical care's complexity, uncertainty, and immediacy are often taken out of the realm of right/wrong and squarely placed into the quest for the best decision. Utilizing the entire triangle of data and process, EI and intuition elevate us into the most favorable situation to make the *best* decision.

Defining an organization's *culture* through the leaders or executives is of utmost importance. This is not a "paste-on" and, despite the parade of outside consultants, does not develop from external change agents or is copied from "top" organizations [(50) Frisina p. 27]. One very respected consulting group spent weeks in one of our hospitals, observing and questioning key staff. They then presented a slick presentation that outlined many ideas for change and improvement. Most of their recommendations had previously been articulated by the internal team and brought to local leaders many times. Although this costly redundancy was recognized, the leadership felt that getting outside experts to validate recommendations would solidify the chances for specific change.

Culture is brutal to measure and harder to have fixed goals. Still, it is at the heart of great relationships with patients and the maintenance of quality and safety throughout the organization. It is also challenging to change.

⤴ The Covid pandemic has tested leadership styles. Rebecca Penty and Bret Begun, writing in February 14, 2022, edition of Bloomberg Businessweek (51), state, "Goodbye Plan, Hello Scenarios" and add, "Ambiguity, unintended consequences, and rapidly changing environments are now the norm, and executives must incorporate new leadership styles" (52). Openness and trust, flexibility, teams, and brainstorming are the essential elements of an *active* rather than a *passive culture.*

⤴ If we didn't realize it before COVID Leadership at all levels needed the ability to reframe our culture from passive to active. Authors such as Boleman and Deal recognized the need to REFRAME, and have leaders look at things from a different angle and approach them in a different manner. (53)

⤴ "Because organizations are complex, surprising, deceptive and ambiguous, they are formidably difficult to comprehend and manage. Our preconceived theories and images determine what we see, what we do, and how we judge what we accomplish. Narrow, oversimplified perspectives become fallacies that cloud rather than illuminate managerial action. The world of most managers and administrators is a world of messes: complexity, ambiguity, value dilemmas, political pressures and multiple constituencies…For those with better theories and the intuitive capacity to use them, with skill and grace, it is a world of excitement and possibility. [(54) Pg. 41]

Changes and challenges daily, confounding the already existing uncertainty and complexity of the hospital environment, cannot be subordinated to words indelibly etched on concrete walls. "The pandemic has shut the door on the value of meticulous planning" (55). On the other hand, active culture can also take full advantage of leadership EI and intuition. When this takes place "on the ground," not at the national corporate office, it also has the added benefit of directly impacting the amygdala and connecting to the staff members ultimately responsible for the action.

The essence of accountability and personal commitment is at the core of the second **W**, or **WHY**. Why are we as individuals working in this environment? We must first understand ourselves and our motivations to be successful. Hospitals, and in general medical care, are primarily a people business. There has been astronomical growth in diagnostic marvels such as the CT scan, the MRI, and the PET scan. These developments have multiplied our diagnostic capabilities many-fold, but perhaps they have partially obscured that health care is still people taking care of people.

If you ask the prototypical nurse why they are in the medical field, they often use the hackneyed statement "they want to help people." Although this is true, Sinek says "that it is primarily the feelings that one gets from belonging to an institution that has shared values, and being around others with shared beliefs that provides the most powerful draw to the organization."

We are attracted to the vision and the mission. This may be plastered on the facility's walls to help us identify with the organization. However, it belies the fragility of the relationship and the need for constant reinforcement. These feelings must be validated constantly with meaningful dialogue, follow-up on issues small and large, and the ability to touch each employee at a limbic or midbrain level. This is not about salaries or recognition, although these certainly help solidify an employee's place in an organization. It is about emotional contact. This contact relies heavily on the leadership role. Like dogs, employees can sense the veracity of their managers and executives and the ability to trust the message and the leaders themselves.

"We are drawn to leaders and organizations that are good at communicating what they believe," writes Sinek [(56) p. 55]. "Their ability to make us feel like we belong, to make us feel special, safe and not alone, is part of what gives them the ability to inspire us. And we feel a strong bond with those who are also drawn to the same leaders and organizations."

Embedded in the many books on leadership (way more than I have referenced) is also a very special skill. Amy Cuddy in her book <u>Presence</u> quotes William Ury:" When you listen to someone, it's the most profound act of human respect" [(57) Pg. 76] As a Leader of many teams and groups I was called to task one day by one of my subordinates. I thought we were having a really good conversation about some specific quality metrics until she interrupted and said, "You are not listening to me". This almost brought me to my knees, since I thought that was in general one of my attributes. I relearned a lesson that day, and hopefully, have been a better leader for it.

Why we are here then depends on a similar triangle of interlocking attributes, as described earlier in the context of decision making. Our attraction and commitment to the workplace are based on three major things. The first, of course, is data-driven and based on benchmarks we have developed during our careers. We want to work and belong to a unique organization. When I presented the fact to employees and managers of one organization that it had reached an A in one national ranking and Five Star in another, the swelling of pride in each individual was palpable.

From our limbic system, the second reason comes from our biases and relies on intuition and all the history and experience it represents. Both Gladwell in *Blink* and Sinek in *Start with Why* discuss people's commitment to working in situations such as hospitals. "The power of Why is not opinion, it's biology," claims Sinek [(58) p. 55]. "The limbic brain is responsible for all of our feelings such as trust and loyalty and is also responsible for all human behavior" [(59) p. 56]. This gut-level feeling of being part of a family contributes to the culture of excellence at some facilities.

There is, of course, tremendous variability in institutions, and the size is often a significant factor in how employees connect. Large hospitals often have multiple silos, and the only feeling of belonging and family comes from specific unit associations. Smaller hospitals may have a more pervasive family culture that crosses over departmental lines.

The last element of this **WHY** is our emotional intelligence and how we connect with our peers, our leaders, and their vision. This is critically important as it affects how we feel about what we are doing and is also based on our personal involvement and accountability. This gut-level connection differentiates an organizational culture that mandates excellence. In the hospital environment, that translates to caring about our patients, listening to what they are telling us, and acting in the patient's best interest over whatever inconveniences or difficulties.

✴ There are two vital elements of this interpersonal connection. The first is understanding at a human level the needs, wants, and capacities of the people you are working with, report to, and interact with professionally. Goleman classifies this under the heading of empathy, which he describes as "sensing others' feelings and perspectives and taking an active interest in their concerns." The second, and more critical, is honestly understanding oneself and recognizing one's emotional state under various situations. This self-awareness is not a slam dunk by any means. It often takes maturity based on a significant underpinning of experience. It takes self-confidence and looking at oneself truthfully. With some ability to do this, we are better equipped to work as a team and better understand the individual needs of our patients and peers.

As described by Richard Restak, the limbic brain is responsible for much of our emotional connections, but it is the MPFC (medial prefrontal cortex) that "springs into action whenever we direct our attention inward and think about ourselves, or outward and think about others" (26: p.72). The limbic system and the prefrontal cortex have been demonstrated physiologically as the neurological elements that house the brain's workings, allowing for human connection.

Having the ability to connect is a positive component of our patient care skills. It is also a necessary piece of our culture. It allows us an enhanced relationship with our patients, but it can also provide us with emphasis and motivation to understand the safety and quality data cascading around us. It is part of what belonging to a high-functioning team makes us feel.

Without this neurological reflex being activated, taking care of patients is just a task. Without this inherent deep-seated activity in the brain, delving into the systemic quality and safety issues, taking *ownership* and doing something about them is increasingly problematic.

Dr. Fields (pseudonym as are all the names in this book) was an orthopedic surgeon who connected with his patients and had the skills to provide excellent surgical outcomes. After many years of the standard approach to knee replacement surgery, he added minimally invasive surgery (MIS) to his armamentarium. There was significantly less cutting of tissue, a smaller incision, and much more rapid recovery in MIS knee replacement. In a couple of his early cases with MIS, the patients developed superficial wound infections, which was unusual for Dr. Fields. When investigated, his infection rate was still well below the national average. He could have treated the superficial infections with antibiotics and been well within the standards of care. However, with the help of the hospital quality and safety team, driven by Dr. Fields' and the hospital staff's accountability for each and every patient, an intensive evaluation was undertaken. Charts were thoroughly reviewed. The patients and treating nurses and techs were interviewed. Cultures were taken of the operative equipment and all items that may have touched the patient. Indeed, cultures were taken from the doctor's nose (which can sometimes harbor infectious germs), and all revealed no contributory factors.

It was then decided to videotape the operative procedures on the subsequent patients (protecting, of course, the privacy of the patient and with their permission). During the review of the cases, it was noticed that, with the extra-small surgical incision, which was the hallmark of MIS surgery, Dr. Fields did a lot of handling and traction of the tissue around the incision with toothed forceps to get adequate visualization, as well as the ability to complete the procedure. The suggestion was made to enlarge the incision slightly to decrease the amount of potential stress on the tissue around the surgical site. There were and have been no further similar infections.

Dr. Fields had to discuss openly and critically his patients with wound infections, not a pleasurable experience for him. In addition, he had to move past his _confirmational bias._ In distinction from a bias that sometimes comes from narrow-mindedness, and limited experience and exposure, confirmational bias comes from commitment and ownership. Dr. Fields had spent considerable time and personal training to learn MIS's new surgical techniques. He had to watch and then participate in proctored procedures by experts at university and teaching hospital locations. He then had to train the local hospital surgical staff in the new techniques and convince patients of the efficacy of the more recent approach. Psychologically this convinced him and committed him to his new methodology.

Daniel Kahneman, in several books, describes Dr. Field's type of bias:

> "Either we jump to conclusions and simply bypass the gathering and integrating information, or we engage in deliberate thought to come up with arguments that support our prejudgment. In that case, the evidence will be selective and distorted: because of confirmation bias or desirability bias. [W]e will tend to collect and interpret evidence selectively to favor judgment that we already believe or wish to be true.
> "[(60) p. 169]

In reviewing his case, Dr. Fields had to move past this confirmational bias to appreciate the need to alter his new technique slightly. He did this in a manner that improved care and solidified his team's relationship with the surgical and hospital staff. His inherent emotional intelligence, his understanding of himself, and his empathy for his team allowed him to move past his bias. In addition, it was evidence of the active culture of the organization that members of the medical staff were encouraged to embrace progress demonstrated at other institutions and make them their own.

The staff had to commit huge time and effort to resolve a problem that statistically was not significant and would probably not cause any ill effects. There would have been no governmental penalties since there were no medical errors and no statically significant elevated rates of complications. However, the surgeon's dedication, transparency, the analysis of the quality and care teams, and trust and communication allowed for the understanding of the issues and the performance improvement activities of the entire operating theater.

Developing a complex active culture that can adjust to change, communicate clearly, listen carefully, and sustain communication and relationships is critical to **WHAT** we are about and **WHY** we are here. It is pretty clear why we would be attracted to this culture. It is also clear why this type of culture is the foundation of excellence, safety, high productivity, low turnover, and other success measures. From our experience with Covid-19, an active culture is necessary, with committed personnel, to survive a worldwide pandemic of epic proportions.

What does it take to get everyone in the organization to embrace an active culture?

- Clearly stated mission

- Effective leadership

- Effective two-way communication

- Respect

- Clarity

- Honesty

- Trust

- Connection

- Personal accountability

- Self-analysis and understanding

Both Goldman and Restak discuss the strength of employees' emotional connection to the organization and each other. As described earlier, the anatomical locations in the midbrain have been identified as the focus of these feelings. The purposeful or accidental creation of a team enhances and provides measurably good feelings, enhancement of communications, an environment for creativity, and an avenue for the creation of *action*.

Covid-19 is a highly publicized cataclysmic event impacting millions of lives. The repercussions on hospitals and health care systems have been enormous. The demands, risk, exhaustion, and demoralizing impact of so many deaths have produced a level of stress that is overwhelming in the short run and unfathomable in the longer view. Acute stress on hospital staff has provoked severe anxiety, worry, and anger. Christy Matta described in The Stress Response (61) and James E. Loehr in Stress for Success (62) that stress comes from a prehistoric "fight or flight" reaction that is heavily hormonal based. Part of most recent medical training considers this reaction, utilizes it to motivate immediate action, and helps develop the many different techniques used to establish self-control. Many of these attributes are part of our emotional intelligence and sometimes help us perform heroic actions daily.

✳   The longevity, the uncertainty and changing demands of Covid, and the mixed messages from our divided society have demanded a much more forceful response to *chronic unrelenting stress*. The impact of this duration of stress has not yet become evident, but we have already seen wholesale disruption of nursing and other hospital resources. The toll of Covid illness and even the isolation for presumed exposure has decimated many nursing ranks. More subtle but no less formidable is the toll of stress on all medical personnel's long-term health and welfare.

Matta and Lohr, in their works, describe multiple techniques helpful in more positively reacting to acute stress, even utilizing it as a vehicle for higher performance and action. As an emergency physician, I appreciate their understanding of our responses to these critical situations and their advice or training programs similar to world-class athletes' training instruction. The reaction to the chronic nature of the current stress pattern requires additional internal and external resources. Staff support services are extremely helpful. Organizational understanding of the need for more time for staff, even during the shortages occurring during the Pandemic is essential. However, these and other resources can be complemented by individual EI and its elements of self-awareness, self-control, and connection.

Hospitals where empathy is intrinsic, not only for patients but for each other; where the team is an essential psychological as well as operational device; where trust and collaboration and communication, on a limbic level, are the daily norm; where leadership is transformational as well as transactional, have weathered the storm of Covid at a much more sustainable level. Our static culture may have prepared us to accept, even if grudgingly, the disruption of direct relationships with patients and made us accept the intercession of technologies. Still, Covid requires an active culture to respond appropriately. We needed a significant dose of trust in each other, empathy, shared emotional reactions, and humanity to survive as caregivers in an active culture-supported environment.

V.

WHAT (WHAT WE KNOW ABOUT OURSELVES, INCLUDING QUALITY AND SAFETY DATA)

As we move from **WHAT2WHY**, the next step is **WHAT2WHY2WHAT**. This third **W** assumes we have the appropriate culture and grit to look at our organization critically. This is not easy or simple by any means. Years of patting ourselves on the back for doing excellent work, and reinforcing each other in this pursuit, have made us less comfortable looking for landmarks or reflections of how well we were doing or the quality of our care. We needed data for an accurate assessment of our work. This is the basis of the third **WHAT** (what we know).

✦ Since the turn of the century, which seems somewhat strange to articulate, relative to a description of modern medicine, there have been significant internal and external forces shaping our world. The *financial pressures* of an "out of control" health care system have led to an entirely new industry of audit and data and their multiple ramifications. This has, in part, been complicated by the unfulfilled promise of the EHR (electronic health record) and its unintended consequences that we now deal with daily.

In the early part of my career, physicians specifically evaluated their performance through introspection. Did I do a good job? Was the outcome of my actions, either directly or indirectly, favorable? This analysis was done frankly with no eye toward patient satisfaction, concern with the utilization and expense of care, nor for the long-term value of what we did. If there was a bad outcome, we generally blamed the situation and the essential underlying health of the patient. "My patients are sicker" was the oft-heard refrain. As alluded to earlier, this has significantly changed in our current iteration of medicine.

Currently, there is a dual quest for the quality and safety of care and how to measure them. These two conditions are spoken of together so often that it might seem that they are synonymous. They are indeed closely related and may be pictured as two overlapping circles. Safe care is a significant attribute of the quality of medicine. Quality and adherence to its elements most usually lead to safe care. How we evaluate these aspects and measure them and self-evaluation are the basis for our third **WHAT**.

How do we define safety, and how do we determine quality? Is the pursuit for each of these the same? How do we measure our success or lack of success? And finally, once we can understand the goal, how do we get there?

Before defining safety and quality and how to measure them, let's test the concepts with our original **WHAT2WHY**. What are the drivers of our motivation for safety and quality? Perhaps common-sense dictates that the overarching goal is wanting to take care of people. That is undoubtedly true, but what is the business case for good care in the modern world? Public opinion, now guided by many publicly reported data streams, is undoubtedly part of it. The desire for the continued growth of medical delivery systems and medicine's apparently attractive corporate structure is an additional factor.

Today, an even more significant driver is the emotional reports of poor outcomes and safety breaches that frequently appear in the lay literature. Additionally, putting the heft into these programs is the government's role in public reporting and their increasing propensity to implement "pay for performance." The current legal system has also enhanced its potential for inflicting significant financial penalties for malpractice and even for poor outcomes. Medical providers and hospital systems have committed to safety and quality for altruistic reasons, but additionally, they are doing this for direct and indirect financial reasons.

For years, we were told that if we just showed people in health care the data, we could change and significantly improve the way we take care of patients and the outcome of measured *quality* of that care. Our initial approach to this was to choose a *process in the stream* of daily health care "tasks" and try to measure if this was being completed effectively. We chose this approach, simply put, because we could do it. We could do a chart review and hope that the documentation in the written record supported a study of a process, or we could audit by direct observation. One can remember folks with clipboards and stopwatches observing our actions as we tried to take care of patients. No matter the methodology, we were looking at *process measures*.

- We did it because we could, given time and resources.

- The data was timely and theoretically actionable.

- The data, however, was not often statistically significant.

- We had little with which to compare the data.

- We wanted to perform better, but what were the standards?

- The data was hard to risk adjust.

- The measure was of the process rather than of the outcome.

There was considerable resistance to the value and applicability of this form of quality data, particularly from physicians. The wealth of their own experience seemed to outweigh the rather humble data streams of this initial quality data. The refrain of "my patients are sicker" was the trump card in a typical conversation when trying to utilize data to impact the care of patients. The relatively small sample size of most of these early data collections did not carry enough power to undermine the depth of a physician's personal experience.

Physicians also carried forward confirmational bias from their specific experiences even when evaluating validated data. A single practitioner, even if phenomenally busy, by the nature of the interactions with their patients, might experience a minimal view of the myriad of potential health care problems.

John Morro was a thirty-seven-year-old patient presenting with swollen glands in the neck (lymph nodes). John worked as an accountant and was quite excited about his coming wedding the following month. His fiancé noted the swelling in his neck, and because it did not hurt him or cause other symptoms, he chose to ignore it for several weeks. Finally, because of her persistence, he went to see his primary care physician. He was treated with a course of antibiotics, and just in case the nodes did not improve, he was referred to an ENT specialist.

John had to stop the initial antibiotics because he developed a severe rash thought to be secondary to a known penicillin allergy. John was taken up by his wedding and the aftermath for the next few months, but because his swollen lymph nodes did not completely disappear, he finally made an appointment to see an ear, nose, and throat specialist. The doctor expressed some concern about the persistence of the lymph node swelling and noted that they were also swollen on the back of his neck and the usual anterior location, so she recommended a needle biopsy. Rather than have a significant surgical procedure, it was agreed to insert a needle into the swollen area and take a sample that day in the doctor's office.

The doctor called John back approximately one week later and told him that the biopsy just revealed some inflammation and prescribed a course of a different antibiotic. John's new wife was unhappy with the medical issues. She talked to her personal physician, who, on the basis of the story, recommended a surgical excision and removal of one of the lymph nodes, a much more invasive and expensive procedure. John understood that the surgical procedure was to be done at a surgical center and would involve getting some type of anesthesia, opening the area on his neck, and removing an entire lymph node. To make it more comfortable, he would not only get a local injection but would get some medication intravenously to minimize pain, anxiety, and discomfort.

After some hesitation, John finally had an excisional biopsy of his left-sided posterior cervical nodes (From the back of his neck). John and his wife spent an anxious seven days waiting to be told the biopsy results. Holding their breaths, they finally heard that he had Hodgkin's lymphoma from the surgeon. Subsequently, John had seen the oncologist and was receiving vigorous therapy for his condition.

Was the long period from initial evaluation and the consequent "suffering" and potential worsening of the situation below the standard of medical care or just suboptimal? John and his wife had consulted an attorney, and the conversations were ongoing. Is this a patient safety issue, or a quality issue, or is this merely a reflection of the uncertainty of medical practice?

Dr. Timothy Platts-Mills and his co-authors discuss the *uncertainty* of diagnosis and its liability (63). Their article tries to weigh overdone, invasive, expensive, and unnecessary testing against the uncertainty of diagnosis, factoring in the expenses and sometimes the risk of specific diagnostic procedures.

If looked at through the lens of *safety* and the consequent risk potential, John's case would be studied with an RCA (Root Cause Analysis), or at least a case review, looking at the medical judgment, the process of care, and the potential liability. Was there a delay or failure to diagnose? If the issue appeared to be primarily medical judgment, the practitioners would be involved in discussions under the auspices of *peer review*. In the review process, the dialogue and recommendations are protected from discovery by state legislation (1157 in California). A very proscribed system of review, involving open discussion by physician colleagues, followed by the classification and recommendations, is utilized. The potential process issues in John's case would be discussed at the multidisciplinary RCA, with attention focused on the delay in the biopsy process, the allergic reaction to antibiotics, the failure to diagnose by needle biopsy, the access to referrals, and issues of informed consent and communication.

When viewing John's case through the Quality lens, the significant focus initially would be based on looking for larger-scale national data. Rather than a single case, we would look at the track record of the individual physician, the methodology of the needle biopsy, the technique and quality of the pathology over multiple similar cases, and the path to system change and general improvement of care.

There has been a gradual understanding that quality data could measure the effectiveness of care for patients. Still, it was recognized that the US health system did not have a good *ratio of value to cost* that put muscle into the collection and evaluation of quality data. This realization was ignited further in the period 1980–1990 by data that showed the error and complication rate of the American health care system was scandalous.

This later focus came to be known as *Patient Safety*. To the credit of the committed people involved in publicizing the faces of numerous individuals who suffered the consequences of medical errors, it started to popularize the subsequent drive for patient safety. These dedicated individuals were able to jump the gap between the medical-industrial complex, the liability industry, and the public by putting faces and families at the forefront of the discussion. Although there is significant overlap between quality and safety programs, there is often a divide, almost a competition for resources and, more importantly, energy.

The government, hospitals, and health care systems started collecting quality data more aggressively in response to the increasing financial and public pressures to adhere to higher standards. There was also growing awareness that improvements would impact efficiency, resource allocation, and financial solvency in the medical system. For the most part, data collection revolved around "abstraction" at first from the paper chart and then from the advancing EHR (electronic health record).

One of the essential themes in this work is understanding the unique aspects of quality and safety programs. This understanding will, we hope, lead us all to a capacity to integrate these programs, not just labeling them together or even administratively putting them under unified leadership, but operationalizing them together to maximize resources and improve care.

Betty Frask, the nurse reviewer in the Quality Department at one of our hospitals, would pore over individual charts looking for pertinent details impacting the patient's care. Half of the charts reviewed in their paper form would fill a three-ring binder. Sitting alongside the binder would be multiple file folders that contained additional materials from even an average hospital stay. Betty's office had boxes and piles of medical records on every surface that would be reduced into data and trends through her laborious efforts. One could barely find Betty in her cubby office because of the piles of charts around her, but she was uniquely suited for this process, having been a long-term nurse with an overarching knowledge and sense of patients and their care. Even more essential than her background was her patience.

It seemed that Betty worked twenty hours a day to get through the piles and boxes, ultimately coming up with crucial kernels of information that could be used to develop trend data and sometimes even improve the care of an individual patient. Betty would often travel to the part of the hospital where a patient was actively being treated or cared for and sought direct interactions with the staff and even the patients themselves. This provided invaluable additional information about each patient and their care, which is not always documented in the medical records.

The measurement of adherence to best practice and standardized process measures, as collated by Betty, became widespread as markers of *quality*. The selection of these markers was often based on an intuitive feel for elements that would characterize and highlight the quality of care in a patient. For example, the timely use of aspirin on arrival to the emergency department of a patient with chest pain and possible myocardial infarction became a surrogate for overall emergency cardiac care quality. The connection between the use of aspirin and the improvement in outcomes in patients with heart attacks has been well recognized. The immediacy of using a baby aspirin, under ten minutes after a presentation to the ED, either chewed or under the tongue, was considered an indication of early recognition of a heart attack that was trackable and reproducible. Percentage compliance could then be collected with relative ease and compared with historical data and, more importantly, with other hospitals.

✶ The measurement of the use of aspirin on arrival to the ED in a patient with chest pain is no longer used as a quality measure but is an excellent example of a *process measure*. Process measures typically are easily measured, the data numerical and collectible, often electronically, and then relatively quickly available to push process improvement activities.

✶ *Outcome data* rather than process data has become the gold standard for measuring the quality of care, but for the most part, it is not available for the individual hospital. Patients that seemingly did well in the hospital met all the standards of care, or even suffered some complications, were discharged and lost to follow-up. Except in the rare health care system that had comprehensive continuity of care, a treating hospital often did not know if their patient succumbed or even was readmitted to another facility.

✶ Outcome data has become increasingly available over several years, particularly in older populations. The CMS (Centers for Medicare & Medicaid Services) now publishes a copious amount of reliable outcome data. But unlike Betty Frask and her audit approach, this outcome data never comes from seeing a patient or a direct review of a chart. It emanates from *codes* submitted to CMS, often quite removed from the time of care or disposition. The primary use of these codes is financial and are the essential elements of the Medicare billing cycle. They also reflect the measurement of the quality of care, resource management, risk stratification, diagnosis quantification, and mortality and readmission outcome measures. The government never actually sees a patient or even reviews the documentation on the medical record. It only looks at the numbers that are reflections of standardized codes. These codes emanate from rigorous definitions and meet extremely complex but rigorous compliance standards.

✓ This *publicly reported data* continues to become increasingly refined, and perhaps surprisingly, CMS (Centers for Medicare & Medicaid Services) has become more interactive with the recipients, such as individual hospitals. For example, we have a very mature data analytics team in one of our markets, prioritizing validation of all data, particularly from outside sources.

In her quest to understand and validate government data as much as possible, one of my analysts, Alice Johnson, had a history of multiple emails and conversations with the fine folks at CMS. One day in a panic, pale and nervous, she came into my office. As a policeman's wife, she usually had a very level and controlled demeanor. For the most part, data analysts are not known to be excitable or emotional about their work. I reacted to her state as one might expect. She handed me a copy of an email from CMS that said "if you have so many questions and comments, I would like to speak to you directly." This email was from the medical director of one of the significant CMS data programs. "What have I done?" she said. When CMS reaches out to you or your hospital, the feeling is of letting the wolf into the hen house. I took the email copy from her shaking hands, and a smile crossed my face (before we wore masks to protect from Covid exposure). "Did you notice how he signed the email?" I spoke. She replied, "It's from the director of CMS." "That's true," I said, "but he signed it 'Paul.' Usually, you don't get only a first name if they call you to the task."

Several days later, my team and I had a very interactive discussion with Paul that was mutually beneficial and illustrated the collaborative attitude of CMS wanting to provide the hospitals with appropriate actionable data. Of course, Alice, our analyst, was beaming the entire time of the telephone call.

✦ Another force impacting quality and safety has been the increasing undermining of *continuity of care* at all care system levels. There is finally recognition that quality and safety are not inhibited by the walls of the acute care hospital. Hospitals are becoming part of health care systems that include hospitals, physician offices, surgical centers and rehabilitation facilities. They also provide increasing coordination across the medical continuum. Although driven by many factors, such as the need to control overall medical spending, much of the thrust for this direction comes from the loss of *continuity* caused by the collapse of traditional private medical practice. A discussion of these factors focuses on the increasing *complexity* of medical care.

✦ ✦ The number of new disease entities currently described is best understood as part of a fractionating of complexes that were once thought to represent a single medical disorder. This is best illustrated in the fields of oncology and immunology. The laboratory is a different world than it was even ten years ago. The unmasking of the *genome*, even of aggressive new viruses, and the ability to understand the immunology of very specific subsets of a disease, such as breast cancer, are merely examples of today's practice. Along with these advances are the specific treatments that they allow. A forty-two-year-old patient that presents with breast cancer no longer gets a standard menu of surgery, radiation therapy, and chemotherapy but has a tailored program based on the genetics of the patient and the cancer type itself. The statistical improvement in the treatment of this disease is undeniable, but it does come with some cost.

As part of her work-based health insurance, Jane Roche, a forty-two-year-old mother of three children, aged eight to sixteen, had a yearly breast screening exam. These had been relatively uneventful for her in the past. Still, this year after waiting over a week for her results, she was finally called by her regular doctor, who recommended a follow-up ultrasound of a suspicious lesion in her left breast. The ultrasound was done, accompanied by a needle biopsy the following week, and again she was referred to her primary care physician for results. The material from the suspected lesion was thoroughly examined, and blood tests from Jane herself. Her doctor finally called her and recommended that she follow up with a surgical colleague for a partial mastectomy and lymph node resection.

This was just the beginning of Jane's journey in breast cancer diagnosis. She was informed about the multiple statistical choices of therapy and then selected a combination of surgical excision, radiation, and choice of chemotherapy. The duration of treatment and the need for follow-up testing and possible complications were also elucidated. During this time, the role of her primary physician, who had been following her for years, was eclipsed by specialists who provided their unique elements of screening, diagnosis, and multiple treatment options.

Jane was overwhelmed by these conversations and not happy with the process. She was scared and upset by the seemingly endless waits from the original screening exam to actual treatment. It wasn't until far into the process that she finally had the opportunity to sit with a physician who seemed to care and had the time to spend with her not only to understand the issues but also to provide emotional support.

Jane's case is not atypical and represents multiple issues that reflect care in the United States and complicate our quest for *patient safety and quality care*. We know that both safety and quality data are just statistical games. The number of errors, or less than favorable outcomes, is related to the number of processes or acts that accompany each episode of patient care. The *quest for zero harm* with the resources that have been committed in the past is probably not realistic. Approaching zero is a more actualizable measure.

In Jane's case, the number of procedures, interactions, choices, and inherent variation in cancer and the patient allows for the statistical probability of error. If we look equitably at these circumstances, the number of events in this health care stream is the proper denominator, rather than seeing Jane's treatment for cancer as one event. Because of all the factors elucidated above, the complexity of current health care challenges us. The effort to ensure Harm reduction and state-of-the-art quality, cannot simply evaluate Jane's breast cancer as one data point but must be evaluated as a conglomerate of hundreds of complex factors that play into her health care course.

This understanding is also applicable to the data on inpatient errors. When a medication error happens during a patient stay in the hospital, we look at that as 1/1 or at least 1/number of days in the hospital. The numerator changes dramatically when you factor in the multiplicity of events/opportunities. If we count every meal the patient is served, every time the patient gets out of bed, every medication, every diagnostic test and reporting, every procedure, every interaction with nursing, PT and other services, the potential for errors leading to bad outcomes, or for incomplete processes enlarges exponentially. The ratio changes dramatically. In approaching zero errors, understanding the complexity and objective steps then becomes a much more realistic and dynamic approach to the issues of safety.

When factoring in complexity there is no elegant mechanism to accurately compare the number of health care events of patients being treated in the hospital or as outpatients today compared with the late 1990s. When you add the additional dimension of an aging population, the addition of multiple diagnostic and therapeutic measures and the variation and inconsistency of continuity, the complexity of reaching zero errors can be better understood.

PATIENT SAFETY VS QUALITY

Despite the complexity and uncertainty of modern medicine, a rational study of it makes perfect sense. Safety and quality are watchwords that are now shouted in newspapers, journals, books, and TV news and talk shows. Safety, or the lack of safety, has claimed center stage. This is probably for a good reason, and the human stories illustrating medical errors are certainly attention-grabbing. They are also the fodder for legal action and often lead to substantial financial settlements. More poignantly, errors cause unnecessary loss of life and contribute to frequently untold damage to families and caregivers. The million dollars plus payments can only scratch the surface of the damage caused by these events.

Marsha Johnson was a forty-seven-year-old patient receiving therapy for the unfortunate diagnosis of leukemia. She had been well until approximately three months prior when she self-diagnosed herself with the flu. She could barely crawl out of bed, and her husband finally forced her to make an appointment with her family physician. On her visit to her doctor, he noted that she was quite pale and got a CBC (complete blood count) following up on a diagnosis of anemia that he felt was most likely. Marsha had her blood drawn the following morning at the neighborhood lab and went home and climbed bed back into bed. She was somewhat startled when later that afternoon, there was a call from her doctor's office asking her to return that day.

In the past, laboratory work was given to her either by mail or by a call from her doctor's assistant within approximately a week. This was worrisome, so she hurried back to the doctor's office.

"Your blood work shows that you have a type of leukemia," the doctor told her after she sat down across from him in his office. After catching her breath, she replied, "What does that mean? And now what?" She was referred to a hematology specialist and told that he would be the one to answer her questions.

As we have seen with several previous patient histories, Marsha was now entering a complex medical system with multiple priorities, complicated by her specific diagnosis's variability, complexity, and uncertainty. Unless medical errors or mistakes or parts of her diagnosis and treatment fall out of statistically acceptable parameters, the data about her care, treatment, and ultimate quality of life may never be measured. Current information about the patient experience is being integrated into the data that reflects the quality of care, but much of this information is mitigated by patient bias and expectations.

The medical-industrial complex is firmly committed to the ideal concepts of *quality and safety*, and it is inherent in the healthcare system culture. This, as mentioned several times over the last pages, was not always necessarily true. Frankly, we were frequently bogged down in our silos and always had the excuse that our patients were unique and sicker. We have been dragged out of our individual "laboratories" and forced to contend with increasingly vigorous local and national data streams. Admittedly, this data reflects what we can measure and cannot be looked at in isolation from the human-to-human context of our care. What we know, reflected in an increasing amount of data, cannot replace the human elements that are, or should be, the backbone of our goals.

The data that is now readily available represents the entire spectrum of care and reflects a worrisome picture of our modern medical world. This data represents the third **W** in our cascade or **WHAT**. What do we know about what we are doing? I have to admit we have gone from the disdain of data, from intense reluctance to accepting the validity of data, to utilizing the data to 'holler' our excellence.

Finally, we are engaged in a vast effort to prioritize the data and understand it. Then the end game is actually being able to improve the data by seriously improving outcomes in our care. It is also important to remember that **WHAT** we know, or the data aspects does not represent the complete picture of humans taking care of humans. There are heavy midbrain and emotional elements that are important but difficult to evaluate that are the substrate of the visible and measurable.

Before diving further into this **WHAT**, it is essential to understand the milieu in which these considerations must be seen. In some manner, it seems counterproductive to leave the focus on data. Still, this approach reflects the need to look at the people involved and their environment before jumping into statistical information and *grades*. The fact that we can produce timely and relatively accurate data on a large assortment of health care functions has the risk of focusing on the way posts rather than the final destination.

No matter how we cut and slice it, the data is only a reflection of what we as assembled individuals are doing hourly and daily. It should go without saying that the information is not only a compendium of what the doctors and other primary providers are doing, it reflects the efforts of a myriad of bedside individuals who often are under a tremendous time and resource crunch. Patient care requires constant management of not only variegated and diverse diseases and traumatic events, but also of the inherent biases that impact our judgment at every level.

Dividing our environment into attributes will help us understand the vicissitudes of human-to-human patient care and the totality of **WHAT** we are about.

To help us focus, a list of "C" words will be discussed in some detail. Perhaps this is somewhat of a word game, but in discussing these factors, it is easier to internalize and understand the essential elements in our culture necessary to achieving our goals.

- Communication

- Collaboration

- Continuity

- Contact

- Context

- Complexity

- Concern/Caring

- Competence

- Certainty (Uncertainty)

- Count (Accountability)

- Compliance

- Consequences

COMMUNICATION

Marsha Johnson, the forty-seven-year-old with newly diagnosed leukemia discussed above, illustrates our dependence on communication. In many studies, when patients are asked about the most critical aspect of their care, it is communication. Patients want the time to ask questions and be heard, including their worries and concerns. They also deserve a translation of the complex medical jargon often used. Despite varying levels of sophistication, language barriers, cultural and traditional misconceptions, and multiple biases, the key to successful treatment is the inherent understanding that the patient and family possess of their illness. This is not just a nicety reflected in the now omnipresent patient satisfaction surveys but is the essential care element.

Marsha not only needed an explanation and discussion from her care provider but had to suffer the delay and the worry and the grief that accompanied it. Unfortunately, it is not unusual for patients to systematically go from physician to physician, test to test, procedure to procedure without the benefit of face-to-face time with a provider or substantial direct conversation.

There are many published reports of patients, particularly older individuals, who clearly neither wanted nor could handle unsettling diagnosis, but most patients want to know. Communication is time-consuming. It isn't easy but is an act of compassion and a key element in developing a treatment plan that is coordinated, patient-specific, and ultimately leads to continuity and compliance.

The current discontinuity of care also compromises the lines of professional medical communication. The basic design of our new EHR (electronic health record) world is the facilitation among the various providers that promote sharing information. This, at best, is a work in progress. There are certainly elements of success. The essential availability of data on inpatient, outpatient, laboratory, and diagnostic testing has enhanced the advancement of an efficient care plan. It has reduced duplication. Before the EHR, it was not unusual for a patient to have many repetitive, often quite expensive, tests, so each separate caregiver could view their diagnostic data. Modern health care computer systems make it possible for many providers on a case to view and evaluate the actual diagnostic information and the physicians' notes on their patients regardless of the source.

A patient like Marsha would have had a primary care provider, a heme/oncologist, a pathologist, a radiation therapist, a hospitalist if she needed acute care hospitalization, and other specialists as her condition and other issues demanded. Without the electronic health record, the ordering, evaluation, interpretation, and communication of results becomes complex, redundant, and confusing to the patient and the care team. The goal was to reduce duplication and delays responsible for the unnecessary expense and often added hardship on the patient and family.

The other potential advantage of EHR is safety. Modeled after systems outside of health care, such as nuclear power and aviation, modern health care systems incorporate redundancy, alarms, checklists, the potential ease of data acquisition, and security. The translation to the highly variable, complex, and uncertain world of patient care has not been without difficulty. Currently, members of the care team are paying a price that is quantifiable in terms of time, resources, and overload. The safety aspects of the EHR are often lost owing to the many ungainly processes that are currently mandated for patient care.

✴ The push to integrate AI (autonomous intelligence) into our world, including medicine, is seemingly unstoppable. In actual practice, although the technology is still incomplete, our reliance on it is increasing daily. This is because simple tasks can be done more reliably through computer-assisted programming than by error-prone human beings. This is particularly true when those humans are overworked, stressed, and pulled in multiple directions with various stated and unstated goals. If this sounds like the modern hospital setting, it is reproduced again and again across the continuum of care in all geographies.

Versions of AI have been in place for quite some time. Algorithms, either on paper or computer-based, or process maps, as they are called organizationally, are utilized daily. They provide organization and simplicity in a sometimes chaotic and time-sensitive world. They can be effective as an autonomous memory device and can somewhat make patient care projections on the basis of statistics and probabilities.

There are many examples of successful AI and related technology deployment, but we get to the "self-driving car." Although elements of this trend exist on the streets today, the concept of a total driverless vehicle has alluded to the great minds in the industry. This is probably more technical than we can comprehend, but there is more to driving than keeping a car at a constant speed, not letting it drift off the road, reading a map, finding a destination, and braking. There is a small ball crossing the street in front of the car, and the anticipation that a driver might have that a child will run out into the street to retrieve it allows for an immediate life-saving reaction. Waiting to brake before actually seeing the child would be too late. Anticipating the unexpected, uncertainty, and variability pushed into our psyche in every driver's education course is the same basis for comprehensive medical services.

The approach to a patient requires understanding their physiology, under-lying medical conditions, biomedical and biochemical imbalances, mental status, time of life, and multiple other intrinsic factors. This is complicated by the patient's presenting disease and/or trauma in the bed, who can always provide the unexpected for the treating caregiver. In their book Managing the Unexpected (64), Weick and Sutcliffe detail the skills and processes necessary to manage complex and uncertain situations on an organizational scale. Pema Chodron examines this on the human side in her essays on Comfortable with Uncertainty. (65) Increasingly because we rely on a simplified AI approach to patients, we treat the unexpected less judicially and handle the uncertainties these patients present less capably.

The focus on the computer-based system and its bells and whistles has become the biggest impediment to patient-provider communication. It has dramatically impacted the actual time spent at the bedside or directly with a patient, but it is often a physical and psychological barrier.

COLLABORATION

As reviewed above, the modern computer in the health care setting has improved collaboration. Consider that the health care model has morphed from a patient's doctor taking care of the whole patient to a system where multiple players are part of a team that routinely shares the responsibilities to care for complex diseases and issues. This introduces the possibilities of numerous caregiver strengths being applied to a single patient and the care plan being facilitated by the whole gamut of expanded expertise. In the ideal setting, collaboration is about the multiple people involved trusting each other, respecting each other's viewpoints and opinions, and sometimes retreating from one's thoughts, intuition, and biases.

Peter Campo came to the emergency department in a fair amount of respiratory distress. He was a fifty-seven-year-old man who was well known to the department with a long history of worsening lung disease. As a young man, he started smoking cigarettes when stationed in Croatia while serving in the army. Despite multiple attempts at quitting, he continued to smoke and developed COPD (chronic obstructive lung disease). He was personally well known to many of the providers in the ED and received, almost immediately when walking through the door, respiratory breathing treatments, intravenous steroids, and antibiotics. "I feel much better," Peter told everyone. His doctor observed him for thirty minutes and, after some discussion with the patient, elected to send Peter home.

During the discharge process, Julie McGovern, one of the senior nurses on duty, said to his doctor with a questioning tone, "Doctor, he often rebounds after treatment and usually gets admitted." There were several possible responses under these circumstances. They illustrated much about the patient and the people responsible for his care.

Response number one from the treating doctor: "I know. He seems to have bounced back well with the therapy this time, and he wants to go home, and I am giving him oral medications, and I think he will do fine."

Response number two: "Nurse, I have seen these hundreds of times, and he will do fine. Sign him out."

✓ Response number three: "I was planning to send him home . . . You probably have seen him before. What did you see or hear that makes you concerned about this decision?"

In a high-functioning ED (Emergency Department), the care of patients is definitely a team sport. The physicians make rapid decisions and are often pulled from patient to patient with a limited time at each bedside. Response number three illustrates the security of the physician, the trust and mutual respect, and the environment that permitted a high degree of collaboration. It also demonstrated the communication and collaboration between individuals in a high-stress environment assisted by their self-awareness and other aspects of emotional intelligence.

It sometimes would take only a few words, even a look or gesture, in a high-functioning team. Still, the milieu of respect permitted caregivers, of multiple job descriptions, to communicate openly and honestly. Nurses, respiratory therapists, radiology technicians, EMTs, and even administrative staff are encouraged to speak out in the ED. In a good ED, this skill is developed from close association, ego limitation, historical trust, and the tincture of time. Peter's story is repeated hundreds of times per day and is not restricted to the ED but is quite apparent in other hospital areas.

There is now a body of published work that transcends the ED experience, and it is most dramatic in aviation, where one of the end products is called crew resource management. It was established after some historical plane crashes were attributed to the traditional hierarchy and lack of communication and collaboration in the cockpit. Despite the presence of a copilot and even a navigator, the pilot's judgment was supreme and not to be questioned, even if it was fatally wrong.

First Air Flight 6560, a Boeing 737-200 crashed on August 20, 2011. Although the instrument landing system and Global Positioning System indicated they were off course, a malfunctioning compass gave the crew an incorrect heading. The first officer made several attempts to show the problem to the captain, but a failure to follow airline procedure and lack of standardized communication protocol to indicate a problem, led to the captain dismissing the first officer's warnings. Both pilots were also overburdened with making preparations to land.

(From Wikipedia)

✓ In the emergency department, the physician may be the team leader, but it is his responsibility and privilege to work, listen, react, and depend on their teammates.

⚹ The *patient* is the most significant team member in the ED or general care situations. Their part in communication and collaboration can be the make-or-break piece of the medical puzzle. This collaboration allows for understanding and cooperation, but it assists the patient in taking significant *ownership* of their body and its maladies. Systems that do not factor in the patient and family in the collaboration of care will undermine and disrupt successful medical alignment.

The importance of the team is not limited to bedside care. Both the work on operational excellence and the contributions to the quality and safety of an organization come from meetings that empower all the team members to share, contribute, question, and support each other. There has been a recent trend in some facilities to reduce the number of meetings and in those remaining to make them "stand up" meetings.

The new science of meetings also includes integrating *hybrid* meetings, where digital communication can bring folks from disparate locations together. The focus for planning these has unfortunately been the size and shape of the table, the number of individuals, and the camera focus (66).

⚹ The current rationale is to discourage long and drawn-out, resource-demanding experiences. This thinking is very valuable in the reduction of instructional or informational meetings. These sessions do not serve any greater purpose than well-expressed and edited emails.

Tinkering with the format superficially can improve the value of some meetings, but that should not be the operational point of concentration. Meetings can be an essential part of team building. The opportunity to reach out and touch colleagues in a problem-solving milieu, even if it is only by Zoom, can enhance the participants' connections, group thinking, communication, and empathy. The meetings must of course be agenized and very focal, with note-taking of the discussed issues that then is ideally distributed to all members of the team.

CONTINUITY

It was commonplace for an entire lineage to be cared for by a single practitioner in the past. My grandfather was seen in the small number of rooms attached to the living quarters of his doctor's home. The smell of these facilities was forever embedded in my memories. I'm not sure if these unforgettable scents were from the cleaning solutions used or perhaps from the brown bottles of medications lining the shelves or even a combination of multiple other factors. I remember this scent because this physician was not only my grandfather's doctor but also my mother's and mine. Now, this is ancient medical history, much like the vignette of the cavemen in the opening pages. Still, despite all the fantastic advancements in medicine, the inherent *continuity* exemplified by this and other stories has been eroded and replaced.

It is not unusual for a hospitalized patient to see five or more physicians or advanced care providers every day as an inpatient. Many patients cannot tell you who their doctor is. Although there is notably more continuity in most clinic or office settings, the inability to see one's own doctor, particularly if they are recently released from another health care setting, such as a hospital, is not unusual.

Advancements in the computerized medical record have certainly added to enhancements in communication but fall short in replacing continuity of care. This is not all about information flow but about the bond between patient and provider: trust and mutual respect, ownership, and caring. Despite our best intentions, it is human nature to have a more meaningful relationship owing to the time spent together, physical contact, and knowledge about the patient, extending beyond the collated computerized data derived from a single focused visit.

The lack of continuity may be most visible in patients discharged from an acute care facility. While hospitalized, these patients were not followed or even seen by their primary doctors for the most part. A significant additional problem, unsolved except for a few dramatic instances, is the unavailability of timely follow-up by the patient's primary physician. Hospital systems have jumped through multiple hoops to provide better follow-up opportunities, including hospital-provided follow-up clinics, follow-up RN phone calls, and even *care coordination across the continuum.*

✗ Realizing the dramatic loss of continuity in the care of many patients, many systems have expanded traditional inpatient resources to bridge the gap, particularly after the discharge of patients from an acute care setting. Expanding the traditional role of a case manager/discharge planner, for example, to follow a patient into the post-acute setting until most clinical and social issues are settled had a significant impact.

✓ This all helps but cannot replace the primary physician following a patient before, during, and timely after an acute hospital stay.

CARING

There is significantly less caring about patients and communication when in-person involvement is minimized. There was much discussion about reducing emotional attachments to patients and their families in medical school, lest it develops too much of an emotional burden. This was probably good advice when the family doctor was, in actuality, an extended part of the family. Today the minimalization of continuity undermines caring and, inadver-
✓ tently, the feeling of accountability and responsibility for a patient's care. Most

providers do a professional job in their care, but many lack meaningful caring for their patients.

✸ It is human nature not to care as much for a patient as a physician if you are only one of an extended team of providers. It is the continuity that supports the human nature of personal involvement and commitment to patients, rather than the very episodic nature of the current practice of medicine. Indeed, what is being described should not be generalized since there are many exceptions to this episodic rule, but the "limbic attachment" to patients has much less chance of development.

This is also true of patients minimizing commitment to their therapy when it cannot be identified and personalized. This is most frequently accomplished in conjunction with specific human purveyors of insight, information, caring and wisdom. This falls onto the principal caregiver.

✸ When put into perspective, one of the frequent complaints that patients have is that their doctor did not seem to care. This reoccurring complaint is commonly associated with short patient care interactions, as frequently happens in an emergency department.

✸ An ED physician's amount of time physically spent with patients is limited owing to multiple factors. These include the increased *documentation* necessary to comply with current rules, the amount of time added to get through the *redundancies*, and the amount of time to adhere to *safety checks*. These all make the traditional hands-on relationship with patients increasingly difficult to establish. In addition, the burgeoning reliance on diagnostic testing rather than on comprehensive physical examination further decreases the "healing touch" that once was the basis of doctor-patient relationships.

The attention needed at the computer has somewhat been characterized by pictures that show a "good doctor" using their computer during time with the patient but facing the patient and looking up from time to time. The "bad doctor "is shown with his back or side to the patient while attending to the needs of the electronic health record.

✕   Telehealth has recently significantly further decreased direct personal interactions. One can sit in front of a screen and talk directly to a patient from their screen without physically being close to or touching a patient. The positive impact of telehealth should not be minimized, particularly during the last two years of Covid. Telehealth has helped protect providers from the unnecessary risk of contagion. It was an essential tool during the horrifying times of many acute care hospitals' when they experienced overwhelmed critical care capabilities. Telehealth has assisted the care of thousands of patients who are unable or limited in their ability to access direct care because of physical incapacities or social restrictions. It has enhanced the expansion of resources dramatically, and during the height of the pandemic, as much as 50 percent of outpatient visits in some settings were through telehealth. This has significantly decreased to under 20 percent in most environments as Covid has had a diminishing impact.

✕   These trends have the impact of de-emphasizing the importance of the human touch and patients' emotional and limbic responses to the feeling of being cared for. These elements manifest in the level of care and communication between the doctor and the patient and dilute the individual caregiver's sense of responsibility and accountability. Perhaps the more significant impact of telehealth comes from the patients' loss of a deep understanding of their current relationships with the health care team. Not feeling cared for undermines their commitment to the care plan. It certainly can impact their trust and hope, which is essential in the doctor-patient relationship.

CONTACT

Is the doctor-patient relationship still necessary in this age of AI, algorithms, massive diagnostic machinery, and distal telehealth communication? Algorithms are a valuable tool in understanding the primary illness of a patient. They are also essential in the mapping of care plans. There have been multiple studies demonstrating the efficacy of well-researched standardized care approaches. They provide safe and very effective care. They help cut through the complexity and reassure that the essential elements and safety measures are effective. They also offer tools for communication for the nurses, medical assistants, physical therapists, respiratory therapists, radiology technicians, pharmacists, and all the other team members involved in the patient's medical care. Algorithms help ensure everyone is on the same page, facilitating data collection since standardization makes assembling process and outcome data more accessible.

✦ *Algorithms* are the jumping-off point for *artificial intelligence*, and as machine learning becomes more and more sophisticated, they are increasingly valuable for our complex medical world. This standardized process also becomes a significant tool in quality and process improvement but cannot or should not replace contact with patients either emotionally or physically.

Perhaps the lack of contact most recently supported by modern methodologies in response to the Covid pandemic puts patients and their caregivers at a disadvantage. Significant barriers were placed on both patients and providers as Covid ravaged our facilities. PPE (Personal Protective Equipment) was a substantial barrier necessary to protect staff and the spread of COVID to other hospitalized patients. The integration of telehealth equipment kept many of us safe but had the unwanted psychological impact of permitting us *not to touch patients.*

Contact, particularly physical contact with patients, is necessary for the other two corners of our patient care triangle to function thoroughly. Emotional intelligence is most apparent when not filtered through complex technologies. Intuition also flourishes when patients' situations can be the stimulus for multiple questions to the doctor or other team members.

Contact is another critical element of the team approach to patient care and should focus all of us on the importance of collaboration. The more fully all the team members recognize that their function is not only following the algorithm, the more fully all the elements of care can best be provided.

Many of the previous examples illustrate how members of a highly functional team are essential to inpatient care. Constructing a team that maintains contact and support for overarching issues at the administrative level maximizes and focuses energy, understanding, and commitment to propagating an active culture. This significantly impacts how effective safety and quality data can be better integrated into the health system.

In the inpatient setting, it is the *nursing staff* in contact with patients that is most important. As mentioned in the discussion of continuity, modern health care is usually administered by a series of physicians, each of whom has allotted only the briefest time frame at the bedside, either examining or talking to patients. By the nature of their on-hand tasks, the bedside nurse has the opportunity to touch patients in both therapeutic and other ways that project caring. Their observations and interpretations are as important, if not more important than their tasks. The nurse's ability to open lines of communication and their sense of *why things are the way they are* in their patients' lives gives them tremendous insight. Their ability to connect on a human level is valuable in understanding the underlying illness and facilitating therapeutic plans.

Mary Smithson was an eighty-one-year-old admitted to an immense tertiary care teaching hospital in a West Coast city. She was being evaluated for intermittent abdominal pain as an inpatient because she was legally blind and lived at home alone. Most hospitals claim that their goal is excellent patient care. Although this is also the goal of a teaching hospital, the secondary goal is to provide education and experience to medical students, residents, and specialty fellows. This secondary goal exacerbates the issues of physician continuity and heavy reliance on diagnostic testing. Much, therefore, falls to the nursing staff and their heightened sense of accountability and ownership of patients.

Ms. Smithson was scheduled for a GI series to elucidate her abdominal pain. In preparation, she received a bowel prep to cause emptying of the GI tract to allow visualization of her small and large intestines. For most of us, drinking thirty ounces of a phosphate liquid would be quite uncomfortable, as it is usually rapidly followed by explosive bowel movements. Complicating this procedure was her blindness and age. Her nurse dutifully assisted her in drinking the liquid, supporting her efforts manually and encouraging words. After scout films showed an incomplete emptying, she was tasked to drink two further huge bottles of the liquid prep. The result was further discomfort from the resulting liquid expulsion from her already painful and sore bottom.

A few minutes after Ms. Smithson's last uncomfortable episode of watery diarrhea, one of the residents tasked her nurse with telling the patient that the test had been canceled. The nurse had had enough and asked the young doctor why. The reply engendered the following dialogue:

Doctor: "We don't really need the test right now."

Nurse: "Are you going to explain that to her?"

Doctor: "No, you can tell her, and when we come by on rounds, we can discuss it further with her."

Nurse: "Doctor, respectfully, do you understand that after the hardships of the preps, in this blind lady canceling the test may have a terrible psychological toll? At her age and condition, do you want her to think no one cares and give up completely?"

Doctor: "It was the attending physician's decision, not mine."

Nurse: "Perhaps I should talk to him directly then?"

Doctor: "No, I will try to talk to him about the concerns about canceling."

✓ It is the nurse and the bedside caregivers that ultimately have the responsibility and accountability for most of the care that is provided. Physical contact with the patient helps, from a very midbrain level, facilitate a meaningful connection. Without this personal connection, the hard work that goes into taking care of a patient, studying the available data and making improvements, being an active team member, and putting oneself squarely in the picture doesn't happen.

The corollary impact of the loss of direct connection to a patient is that the emotional dividends delivered to the staff from all their good work are also not as available. Part of **WHY** we are here, discussed in the initial chapters, is because of this very limbic feeling of satisfaction. This does not require a "thank you" but tracks back to the gut-level response we get from taking direct care of patients.

I just finished a preview of a keynote lecture at a national emergency medicine conference. A significant part of the theme was the overwhelmed position so many of our caregivers found themselves in during the Covid pandemic. Struggling with the incredibly nasty illness, with so much uncertainty, the personal risk, and the frustration of losing so many life and death battles caused enormous "burnout." In the face of this real-world crisis, a ridiculously few caregivers left the fight, many of whom stayed at their posts, suffering severe physical and emotional harm. In part, this came from professional commitment and, in some cases, even financial incentives. Still, for the overwhelming majority, it came from a deep-seated *midbrain connection* to the plight of patients and the needs of their coworkers. Holding a patient's hand, even with gloves, mask, and gown, provided patients with significant comfort and was terrific to watch. It must be recognized that direct contact fuels the fires at the core of the caregiver's existence.

CONTEXT

The upgrades available to our diagnostic and therapeutic quivers are amazing. The impact of computer programs, technology, and medical breakthroughs such as the Covid vaccines has changed the landscape of medicine forever. They help us, with laser-like focus, deal with our patients. However, they should not replace or invalidate the understanding of the context of our patients. It is not that we currently repudiate the need to take an excellent history of the patient presenting with a headache to the emergency department. Understanding who brought the patient to the ED, the emotional reaction of family members, the cultural venue, and the patient's deepest fears and concerns is essential to understanding the patient's symptom complex. In addition, we needed to comprehend what were our own caregivers' personal biases about headaches and the need for pain medication. Other issues included how busy the department was, which nurse was taking care of the patient, and multiple other factors.

Rocky Jeffries was a thirty-two-year-old male presenting with a severe headache to the emergency department. He had been treated three times over the last several months in the ED, with a diagnosis of headache of uncertain etiology. After getting the patient in a bed, the first thing the staff did was to check CURES (controlled substance utilization review and evaluation system). The primary purpose of this program is to maintain a database that limits the overuse of opioids in either patients or physicians. Many patients will shop around from doctor to doctor or ED to ED looking for narcotics. The program has significantly impacted the overuse of controlled substances

Mr. Jeffries was treated with painkillers after a negative CT scan of his head showed no abnormalities. After his CT scan was negative, a brief reexamination revealed that Rocky continued to be in significant discomfort. The patient's wife was very adamant about needing further immediate pain relief and was very overt in her demands to the ED staff. The ED physician was called out several times while examining Rocky to see other more extremely ill patients (Statistical data from busy emergency departments show the ED doctor is interrupted about every six minutes.). The patient was given intramuscular opiates and demonstrated significant relief of symptoms. Shortly after that he was sent home and told to follow up with his primary care provider.

The treatment and disposition of this patient were complicated by significant bias. This patient was neither of color, homeless, unkempt or jobless. He spoke English as a primary language and had no evidence of substance abuse.

However, there were multiple biases in play that directly or indirectly affected the outcome of Rocky's care.

✦ The patient's family was loud and disruptive in the waiting room, as their non-emergency status was confirmed at registration. Even in a busy ED, this behavior usually sends a ripple through the staff, even when not directly experienced by the caregivers ultimately caring for Rocky. Owing to space limitations during a hectic time in the ED, complicated by mandatory Covid restrictions, the patient was placed in one of the outer rooms of the department. The patient's wife interpreted this placement as the staff underestimating the importance or seriousness of Rock's symptoms. This accelerated her already anxious behavior, complicated because no specific diagnosis was made on his previous two ED visits.

These elements only further polarized the situation. As the ED doctor entered the room, he was immediately met with hostility and distrust, and he responded with concern that the patient had not followed up with referrals made during his last visits. His effort to examine the patient was met with increasing anxiety on the part of the family about treating the patient's severe headache. Relying heavily on Rocky's negative CT evaluation and the demands of multiple other really sick patients in the ED, the order for IM pain control was embraced by the family and care team.

Be assured that Rocky did fine in both the short and long run, but his care illustrated several essential aspects of modern health care.

The family bias based on previous ED experience significantly impacted the communication and collaboration of the ED care team and the patient and family.

1. The context of the less critical room choice, understandable in the circumstances of a busy ED, intensified the family's anxiety.

✓ 2. The ED doctor and team had a significant bias about the demand for opioid pain control in the face of the newest recommendations and restrictions on opioid use.

3. There was an overwhelming reliance on diagnostic technologies to rule out serious underlying medical issues.

4. There was a disabling of the emotional intelligence and intuition of the care team due to the fear and anxiety created by the unruly and disruptive patient and family.

5. The ED physician's bias was. perhaps appropriately, the pressing need to deal with the Emergency Department's "sicker" patients.

6. There was a failure to connect with the patient on a limbic level and the secondary lack of empathy was demonstrated to the family only intensifying their anxieties.

A different set of circumstances would have perhaps revealed that the wife's uncle had recently died of a brain tumor. Having the opportunity to examine the patient even briefly might have developed a human bond that would have enhanced the connection and communication and certainly would have been significantly more evidence to the patient and family of the team *caring*.

Reliance on the advanced diagnostic capabilities of the CT scan to better understand the physical status of the intracranial space and brain has advanced our understanding of the nature of headaches and the ability to rule out severe markers of disease. This approach is considered part of the "gold standard" of care. How to weigh the need for a CT, which is costly and resource-heavy, in the numerous patients with headaches presenting every day to the ED has been statistically studied, but it does not answer the question in a single patient at a time of evaluation. What hopefully is more apparent is the need to understand the context of a patient both from the patient and staff point of view and how family bias and staff bias can play a significant role in patient care, not just in finding the correct diagnosis.

COMPLEXITY

The discussion of safety in the medical world has often been compared with aviation, particularly military aviation, and the nuclear power industry. Catastrophes in those areas have substantial societal impact, loss of lives, and far-reaching consequences. However, every year, those in medicine have hundreds of thousands of deadly events that far outnumber all other industries.

Our goal of significantly reducing these events and the mechanism of how to achieve that will be discussed more in the coming chapters. We are not dealing with diagnoses or therapies but with individual patients and their responses. Patient-focused statistical complexity and its evil twin *uncertainty* up the ante considerably when trying to squeeze out the meaning of individual safety events. Most industries control complexity and uncertainty by simplifying, standardization, practice, and redundancy.

Nuclear power and aviation have phenomenally successfully reduced risk and safety events through these factors and the watchdog capabilities of finely directed computerized programs. Applying these practices in patient care is much more complex when the time demands of emergency and urgency are added to the mix.

> As spoken by an intensivist, "I can't manipulate order-entry fast enough to keep up with the demands, factoring in the changes and uncertainty of direct patient care."

Most critical care doctors would rather have a scribe or a medical assistant enter the documentation, respond to alarms, and make timely adaptions to the vicissitudes of each patient's unique individualized needs. This, of course, reintroduces the potential impact of the game of telephone we played as kids. The number of individuals in a circle passing information significantly increased the aberrant nature of the final articulated message.

More time facing the computer screen and following the programmatic rules means less time at the bedside communicating, examining, and allowing the trained senses to work. The impact of computer-generated health care also adds a significant reduction in satisfaction for the caregiver. It is a great tool that we, as a culture, have committed to, but it decreases our connection in general and certainly at a midbrain level.

Advanced programs will continue to evolve that at least statistically factor in the complexity and uncertainty of our patients. Artificial intelligence and its advances promise machine learning to adjust for these factors but cannot replace the human application of intuition and emotional intelligence.

Newer care providers, who have never functioned without a computer at their elbow, will continue to demand upgrades that favor quicker and more specific methodology. This is excellent news, but it only underscores our increasing reliance on technology and implicitly undermines the additional impact that intuition and emotional intelligence provide.

We must strive for a *balance*. There are far too many errors in our world. For the most part, these errors are not from a lack of knowledge or poor training and development. These errors occur at all stages of experience in caregivers, from the newbies to the nearly retired to those at the top of their game. Dr. Atul Gawande has written about and done much to highlight medical errors. He believes "we need a different strategy for overcoming failure, one that builds on the experience and takes advantage of the knowledge people have and makes up for our inevitable human inadequacies. And there is such a strategy-It is the checklist" [(67) p. 13]. Published almost thirteen years ago, his advice has, in many ways, become one of the mainstays of our computer-assisted intelligence system.

In the face of complexity and uncertainty, the *Checklist Manifesto* falls somewhat short and potentially undermines personal accountability. As Pema Chodron says, "We can try to control the uncontrollable by looking for security and predictability, always hoping to be comfortable and safe. But the truth is that we can never avoid uncertainty. This not-knowing is part of the adventure" [(68) p. 5]. Covid-19 has undoubtedly provided a significant share of uncertainty. The morphing virus, the changing rules of isolation and care, the variability of the response of our communities, the anti-vax movement, and the questionable validity of data made hospital planning even a week in advance nearly impossible.

Checklists, the computer-based EHR (electronic health record) , and even AI cannot eliminate uncertainty as it advances. In some ways, the flip side of this adventure demands even more from caregiver personal *account-ability*. It also helps to understand the midbrain drive in many caregivers to run toward the unknown, the critically ill, and the uncertain. This provides a tremendous feedback loop to caregivers in the emergency department, the intensive care units, the trauma facilities, and high-risk OB and related specialties. High risk, to be sure even high drama from time to time, but the inherent *amygdala* feedback loop provides enormous satisfaction and feeds the fires of personal accountability.

(A)COUNTABILITY

Hopefully, you will forgive me for adding accountability to our "C" list for discussion purposes. Much of the thesis of this book is that *personal account-ability* is one of the critical elements of quality and safety in medicine today.

Modern medicine has definitely become a team sport. Many hands are involved in the care of each person, in the hospital, in the clinic, and across the continuum. Although recognizing the increasing need for TEAM in our complex world, the result is that reliance on it threatens the continuity of care. This is particularly true in patients with chronic disease, as dependence on the team may undermine communication, trust, attachments, intuition, emotional intelligence, care plans, and personal accountability.

The bond between the caregiver and the patient is frayed because of these circumstances. In addition to what the lack of continuity does to patient care, it emotionally unties the attachment between provider and patient. The pictures in all the brochures of health care systems show the hand-holding of a patient and the bedside caregiver. When does that happen routinely with a doctor the patient has only met briefly, amongst the panel of several doctors and specialists, and the nurse assigned four patients/shift and works three days per week? When does that happen in the clinic or private office setting when a patient might encounter the front-end people who do registration, the medical assistant, the office nurse, the advanced care provider, the primary doctor, the discharge folks, and multiple others as well? When does a bond get established, which is necessary to develop accountability? If the only push toward responsibility is the fear of making a mistake and getting into a legal quagmire, as Dezi from the I Love Lucy Show would say "we may have some serious 'explaining' to do, Lucy."

COMPLIANCE

Compliance is another fundamental factor in our world. Many of the surveys by governmental and specialty organizations that focus on the quality of care and the safety of our patients inspect primarily for compliance with the existing thousands of *rules* and *regulations*. It is an enormous task and done exceptionally well by The Joint Commission (TJC), on a national level and by state and local agencies such as the State Department of Health.

Hospital accreditation standards are contained in a book thicker than the old-fashioned phone books some of us grew up with—the following lists just a representative few of the graded standards.

- EC-1 Environment of care

- EM-1 Emergency management

- HR-1 Human resources

- IC-1 Infection prevention

- IM-1 Information management

- LD-1 Leadership

- LS-1 Life Safety

- MM-1 Medication management

- MS-1 Medical staff

- NR-1 Nursing

- RI-1 Rights and responsibilities of the individual

- SEI-1 Staffing effectiveness

The above and other standards are measured on a three-point scoring scale: Insufficient Compliance gets a 0, Partial Compliance receives a 1, and Satisfactory Compliance gets a 2. This vigorous TJC process may have five or more surveyors representing different specialties and may spend as much as a week or more in person at a facility. The certificate of compliance with standards is issued for two to three years, and then the process begins again.

Surveys and the successful designation of a provider, clinic, or hospital are focused chiefly on compliance. Laudable goals, reaching full compliance, but it is not an avatar for excellent patient care. Compliance with TJC or other rating agency standards cannot measure the connection to our patients and the resulting accountability, ownership, and limbic gut-level involvement in care at the bedside.

Our current care milieu and the need to focus on compliance may further undermine the connection between caregiver and patient. Too many obstacles stand between the patient and the care team members. Some are very obvious, such as the attention and demands of the electronic health record, which stands firmly in the middle of all current therapeutic relationships. Some of these disruptions are caused by the intermittent presence of many caregivers in any one case. Some are fiscal and operational demands that factor into the timing of care, the length of care, and the approval for care that are increasingly decided by government or private insurers. Behind all of these demands is the constant push for more and more documentation, which becomes the focus of care rather than the patient.

I have beaten this repeatedly about documentation because it often negatively impacts a patient's care. Still, my focus in these paragraphs is on the impact of the care provider and the gut feeling of accountability that they possess.

Factoring all these forces and the reliance on TEAM is complicated, but at the midbrain level, it undermines connection, accountability, and, unfortunately, feelings of accomplishment.

COMPETENCE

Professional competence is assumed in doctors, nurses, airline pilots, and nuclear safety engineers. Yet intrinsic to their roles, they are responsible for *human error*. No matter how intelligent, well trained, or even experienced, no matter how focused or your usual attention to detail, there is a statistical probability that a mistake, error, or omission will occur shortly.

Much of the subtext of this book is that the more you care, <u>the more you are connected, the more</u> <u>accountable and the more ownership you feel</u>. The engineered process reduces the risk of human error but perversely also minimizes the role of human competence. When the checklist replaces critical thinking rather than assisting it, dependence on it will ultimately erode our capabilities and long-term competence.

(UN)CERTAINTY

Bobby Tailor was a twenty-eight-year-old male presenting to the emergency department with persistent pneumonia. Bobby was a rising set designer in Hollywood but had been unable to work for several weeks because of his declining health. Previously, Bobby played soccer on the weekends with a group of friends and often partied in the local evening scene. Hence, his latest physical ailments were new and totally unexpected. When seen by the doctor in the ED, he related a history of good health, no travel out of the United States, no known exposures, and no allergies. A chest X-ray showed patchy infiltrates bilaterally consistent with pneumonia, most likely viral. He was sent home on a course of oral antibiotics and told to follow up with his doctor. Neither he nor the ED Team worried about him because of his age and essential good health.

Ten days later, he returned to the ED for a further decline in his health. Being young and previously healthy, he did not have a regular doctor to follow up. In this presentation to the emergency department, it was clear that he was sick. He had lost weight and had dark circles under his eyes and a sallow color. An additional X-ray revealed a worsening of his pneumonia. The doctor noted a single purplish skin lesion on his face, and when questioned about it, the patient claimed that he had just recently noted it. When examined more carefully, Bobby admitted that he was frequenting the bathhouses in Los Angeles. Because of his deteriorating health, he was admitted to the hospital but with an uncertain diagnosis.

Bobby Tailor died several weeks later from an unrelenting disease. The year was 1981, and he died from a newly recognized disease initially thought to be related to the bath houses somehow, finally diagnosed as a severe immunodeficiency syndrome, associated with pneumocystis pneumonia, an opportunistic infection, and Kaposi's sarcoma (the purplish skin lesion he presented with), called *AIDS* (HIV-1).

Although we got better at the diagnosis and risks of AIDS, it was many years of uncertainty and heartache before we understood the disease and much longer before antiviral medications were introduced that could halt its relentless course.

Several researchers made significant contributions to the understanding and treatment of AIDS patients. Still, it was a tough time of uncertainty and potential risk for those of us in the trenches. A short time later, a known AIDS patient was brought to the emergency department with a severe tongue laceration after a seizure. His tongue was bleeding badly, and every time he opened his mouth and tried to speak, there was a spew of blood droplets everywhere.

✷ Double gloved and suited up with a mask and shield—basically, in a body condom—I sutured up his laceration, with the patient gamely trying to be as cooperative as possible. I had a young family at home at the time, and it was months before I felt perfectly safe. It was many years ago, but I remember the *uncertainty* well.

✷ Our current pandemic has brought back some harsh memories of Bobby Tailor and scores of patients like him. Covid-19 has challenged our health care system severely. Our colleagues in New York fought an initial battle in New York against the virus, uncertain about almost all aspects of its course, treatment, and self-protection. Their heroism under the vilest circumstances reminds us that our world is full of uncertainty, variability, and complexity.

James Gleick in his book <u>Chaos</u> says," The paragon of a complex dynamical system and to many scientists, therefore, the touchstone of any approach to complexity is the human body. No object of study available to physicists offers such a cacophony of counterrhythmic motion on scales from the macroscopic to the microscopic." [(69) Pg 279] Add to this the impact of Covid-19 only further revealed how an active culture is necessary to adapt to the vicissitudes of health care. Despite the advances in technology, it often falls on people to make the right decisions and empower their actions to save lives.

CONSEQUENCES

This section is mostly a wrap-up of the previous pages to better understand the "Cs." I am certainly not making a case to abandon the phenomenal advances in technologies that have changed our diagnostic and therapeutic success. I am not even criticizing the computer's complex world in medicine, the many advances in cross-community communications, the reduction in redundancy, and the apparent safety features embedded in the system. However, the decrease and almost total elimination of continuity across the continuum and the detachment of the caregivers emotionally significantly undermines care. The other side of this same coin is the impact on the caregivers themselves. The reduction in the limbic level of satisfaction with what they do and the decrease in the emotional rewards are a terrible cost.

In the coming chapters, the vast amount of data that is now available that we look upon to improve the care and safety of our patients may have significantly less impact than it should. This is due to the increasing number of barriers or filters between the patients and caregivers. These standardized technologically supported walls now undermine the personal accountability and emotional involvement that we should feel between the care team and those under our care.

VI.

THE DATA IN THE THIRD W: WHAT

Much high-powered statistical data on quality and safety has come in the last decades. Before this period, data was predominantly regional or even local and often hospital specific. There was virtually no data to follow outpatient care, which makes up most of what we do, based on volume. Data collection was significantly impacted by the practitioner's refrain that "their patients were sicker." The direct comparison of outcomes in patients with a heart attack from a rural medical center to an academic tertiary care center stimulated legitimate complaints. Safety and quality data are often lumped together, and indeed there is significant overlap. Still, we will look at them separately and compare and contrast the data streams, the impact, and the opportunities these data sources present.

There is some risk in focusing on individual data separately instead of understanding it as only one step, although an essential one in the overall improvement process. Grades have become national standards, publicized, debated, and used to document clinical success and safety. However, understand that the published letter grade, much like a grade on a paper written in college, should not be the total reflection of a student's knowledge or effort.

It is often attaining a grade or a score that is the corporate or executive goal because of what it means as a marketing tool, its contribution to fiscal stability, or even what it can mean for an organization's ability to fundraise.

Realistically, it is also often a mirror to the individuals providing the care, and this effect should not be underestimated.

Statistically sound results, rather than an endpoint, should be seen as doorways to opportunities for improvement, and as such, they are precious. They should be at the beginning of the conversation about safety and quality, not the endpoint.

✓ The two main types of data we deal with are *process* data and *outcome* data. What percentage of patients arriving at an emergency department with a presenting complaint of chest pain will get an EKG within the first ten minutes of arrival?

John Murphy was a sixty-two-year-old man with a history of cigarette smoking and moderate alcohol (mostly beer) use. He was up in the morning getting ready for work as a foreman at a building site when he felt nauseated and sweaty. He tried sitting and sipping his morning coffee, but after about ten to fifteen minutes, he alerted his wife about how he was feeling. He also told her he was feeling some vague chest discomfort that he rated as a two on a scale of one to ten. After a verbal battle about the next steps, she prevailed and drove him to the hospital, where the triage nurse immediately evaluated him, placed him on a gurney in a treatment room, and told him to undress. An immediate EKG was ordered, and per protocol, the patient was put on oxygen, and the nurse started an intravenous line. According to the computerized time stamp, he received his electrocardiogram seven minutes after arrival at the ED.

✓ The treatment recorded and the timing of the EKG are the measurement of a process that reasonably reflects one of the elements of quality of care in patients with acute myocardial infarction. It is suggestive of the effectiveness of the triage operation in the ED. How much time did a patient spend in the ED before being seen by a triage person to assess the potential severity of their complaint, recognize it, and not delay the care of the patient? It is an indirect measure of how sensitive the front-end folks in the ED are to a suggestive history of heart problems and how quickly, even in a busy emergency department, they can get the arriving patient into a bed for evaluation.

This data also represents how rapidly a fundamental test such as an electrocardiogram can be done. Did the team wait for paperwork and wait for staff assigned to other duties to break away and complete the task?

Alice Baker was a seventy-two-year-old housekeeper who has not felt well for several days. She felt weak and a little dizzy but ignored her symptoms. She denied having any chest pain. That evening her granddaughter came for a visit and was worried about Alice's general demeanor and lack of her usual folksy style. Alice assured her granddaughter that she would contact her primary care doctor in the morning if she wasn't feeling any better. Because of her age and departure from her usual state of health, her granddaughter insisted she is seen that evening, and she drove her to the local emergency department. Alice was placed in a room by the triage nurse and waited to be seen by the ED staff.

An EKG was ordered about twenty minutes after her arrival when evaluated by the nurses and doctors on duty. This patient typically would not fall into the EKG (Electrocardiogram) time process measurement criteria because she denied having chest pain. Alice ultimately was diagnosed with acute myocardial infarction and rapidly underwent a PCI (percutaneous cardiac intervention). She eventually did reasonably well, although there was evidence of heart damage typical of females with heart attacks because of the atypical symptoms not initially alerting the patient to the seriousness of the symptoms.

The measure of the time to EKG is undoubtedly not a measure of all patients' total acute myocardial care while in the ED or of the hospital experiences as a whole. So why do we use it? The main reason, other than that it is a single representative of ED cardiac care, is that it is *easily measurable*. It is internal data specific to a patient that can be retrieved from time stamps on the EHR. It is not subjected to bias and interpretation. It either is or isn't. It doesn't rely on outside sources to provide the data, and perhaps the best reason is it is timely and easily retrievable. It is reviewable from each patient, each hour, and each day and valuable in "fixing" delays that directly impact patient care. Apropos of the staff taking personal responsibility and accountability, this data is attributable to individual staff and available for immediate feedback.

When looking at this data, one has to be very careful to put it into perspective with the hundreds of other process points that make up the total care of a patient with AMI(Acute Myocardial Infarction). However, the data is helpful in the overall improvement process and serves as gut-level feedback that directly touches the staff.

For the most part, much of the process data has traditionally come from the individual hospital or a hospital system. It is quite helpful to have data from multiple facilities to compare. Carrying that data forward to the providers helps underpin the validity and the overall impact.

Quality data traditionally was teased out of the operations of an individual hospital. This was done manually through direct observation and endless paper chart review. There was minimal data exchange, even with geographically proximate facilities. The barriers were the privacy of the individual patients and the hospitals themselves. There was a significant reluctance toward data sharing since it had some potential impact on financial competition between health care facilities. Meaningful national data could be found in professional journals but had less visibility and limited impact.

Data acquisition in the last few years has changed dramatically. Meaningful data increasingly appeared on scorecards from the individual hospital and then was collated with information from the hospital system. There continued to be significant improvements in the reporting of data, but for much of it, it was still many weeks to months old. It was quite helpful to compare hospitals in a system with each other, but sometimes the message was clouded by the lack of statistical relevance. Hospitals with hundreds of patients in a category were compared to those with scant participants, yet the final numbers were comparatively published anyway.

✓ Most recently, increasing data meets *rigorous statistical testing*, and the results allow for meaningful comparisons of the care at one hospital with the patient care of another. As hospital systems have continued to enlarge and encompass multiple geographies and types of hospitals, this statistically significant rigorous data becomes very helpful in defining quality.

Currently, data is available from the corporate office of many different systems and reflects primarily process measurements. Data has become increasingly available electronically from patient charts, which provides timely data, a non-reliance on coding, and an expanded ability to follow up on specific patient care issues.

The expansion of national data sets such as CMS (Centers for Medicare & Medicaid Services) Star Ratings has markedly enhanced meaningful and actionable data flow. The government has become a partner in data acquisition on a massive level, and in cooperation with private organizations such as Leapfrog, national statistically tested information continues to evolve. Programs such as value-based purchasing reflect data that becomes the basis for financial rewards and penalties. Once the purview of limited experts, this data has become increasingly timely, validated, and somewhat surprisingly open to discussion between CMS and other rating agencies, with clinical people at the local levels.

Most facilities now have a vast amount of process-driven local data sets and vociferous amounts of national outcome data. In some senses, it is like "drinking from a firehose," and organizations are challenged to have the methodology and the resources to react to the data. Organizations effectively manage this flow of data and then utilize it for performance improvement. It is a constant quest. In addition, it is integrated into operations and meaningfully incorporated at a limbic level in the staff. This requires significant commitment.

Before a meaningful discussion about the process and outcome data, *social determinants of health* must move to the front of the conversation. This is particularly true if quality and safety are looked at through the lens of continuity of care across the continuum. Social determinants have always played a significant role in health care. Still, the issues of inequality, drug and alcohol abuse, severe psychiatric illness in combination with complex medical presentations, and homelessness have intensified their impact. When looking at performance improvement, these social issues make focusing on PI (Process

Improvement) very difficult. The problems brought to the fore by these issues confuse effective evaluation methodology for many patients.

Max Halter was a thirty-seven-year-old who initially presented to the emergency department with severe blood-tinged vomiting. Max's history was clouded by the fact that he was dropped in the ED by the police, no friends or relatives came forward, and Max himself was either reluctant or unable to provide a past medical history. On arrival, he was unkempt, toes protruding through broken shoes, and had the overwhelming odor of urine on his filthy clothing.

He was very uncooperative, took a swing at his bedside nurse, and had to be put into soft restraints to be examined. The patient had an extremely tender abdomen and was clearly malnourished.

Mr. Halter's evaluation in the ED revealed significant liver disease, pancreatitis, and an alcohol level three times the legal limit. He was initially treated with intravenous fluids, vitamins, and empirical antibiotics because of the suggestion of intraabdominal infection. On day two of hospitalization, he demonstrated severe alcohol withdrawal, and despite appropriate measures, he required sedation and intubation/ventilation for five additional days. After ten days in the ICU with a diagnosis of resolving pancreatitis and liver failure, Max was ready for discharge from acute care.

The previous complicated medical and therapeutic history was the easy part. Patients require a safe discharge before leaving an acute care facility, both morally and legally. Because of his status and history, Max was not a candidate for a liver transplant. Because of his chronic alcoholism and behavior issues, none of the twenty-five SNFs (skilled nursing facilities) connected would consider him as a patient. Although he was found to be a veteran during the later stages of his acute hospitalization, the VA (Veterans Administration) had no appropriate available facilities for his care. A suitable rehab facility finally accepted his care, and the patient was transferred by ambulance. Three days later, Max signed out AMA (against medical advice) from the facility and was initially lost to follow-up. Less than one week later, he was readmitted to the hospital with an almost identical story, and thirty-nine days later, despite supportive care, he succumbed to the complications of his liver failure.

✤ Max's story is reasonably representative of a challenging group of patients. Not dwelling on the social ills in our current society that complicate and may even cause some of his issues, from a quality and safety point of view, makes using only outcome and process data to understand opportunities for improving general care difficult at best.

✤ A growing percentage of medical services are dedicated to the group mentioned above of patients. The hospital-based medical system was not designed to efficiently and effectively handle the challenges these populations present. Consequently, as discussed above, the data derived from care in these groups can significantly skew the interpretation of quality and safety performance.

✤ There are multiple contributing factors to the difficulties in caring for patients with complications from their social situations, but four are the most common: inequality, drug and alcohol abuse, psychiatric illness, and homelessness. Many of these issues overlap in individual patients, further complicating their care.

1.   Inequality

The definition of inequality often depends on the bias of the discusser. This inequality is often an issue because of skin color, language, origin, religion, living situation, financial manifestations, and even body habitus. These patients often face not only the issues of bias but real barriers to effective care. As in Max's case, his severe and relatively end-stage medical conditions were challenging to manage, but they were not only caused by conditions outside of medical control but inherent inequalities of complicated case management. Max's case does illustrate that many of the inequalities of care come from self-inflicted circumstances with long-term consequences. Consider, however, if Max had a family with resources early in his long slide to end-stage health, the possible different resources that could have been dedicated. Many patients like Max had multiple attempts of reintegration within their existing families, but because of severe psychosocial issues, he was ultimately thrown out of his family unit.

2.   Drug and alcohol abuse

It is really outside the scope of this work to discuss how we, as a society, are now embroiled in a fight to survive the widespread use of alcohol and drugs. It is a rare evening news program that doesn't highlight tragedies that have impacted communities because of the direct and indirect use of heroin, cocaine, methamphetamines, and, even more recently, Fentanyl (used as an excellent drug for anesthesia and procedural sedation). The role of big pharma in the string of circumstances that led to widespread addiction to oxycodone and secondary descent into heroin use is not only in the headlines, but is now the subject of docudramas.

Addiction and its effects on patients, families, and society have accelerated the development of in- and outpatient addiction programs with modest success. What is less publicized is the creation of accelerated medical issues in a previously healthy age group. As with Max's case, it impacts not only patients and their families but also care facilities and national statistics. It is disturbing to see members of future generations dying premature deaths caused directly by the medical complications of drug and alcohol abuse.

3.   Psychiatric illness

Suppose you ask the folks in the emergency departments at hospitals across the United States what are the most problematic patients to care for. They will share with you that the percentage of patients with severe psychiatric disease has mounted steadily over the last five years, especially during the pandemic. It is not a surprise that psych disorders have climbed in response to the stress and the consequential circumstances of Covid-19. What actually might be more troubling is that before the pandemic, the number of cases in emergency departments was growing dramatically. This trend is due to multiple factors.

Better recognition of a wider variety of psychiatric disorders.

- More enlightened acceptance by patients and society of the fundamental nature of psychiatric disease.

- Association of psychiatric disease with the two plagues of alcohol/drug abuse and homelessness.

- Outpatient management of even the most serious psychiatric disorders.

- Outpatient management of psychiatric disease was improved by the success of newer, more effective pharmacological agents. In part, this and fiscal concerns caused the consequent closure of state and private psychiatric inpatient facilities.

- There has also been more frequent use of multiple mind-altering medications that may have a worsening effect on psychiatric symptomology and side effects.

Not only are there significantly more psychiatric cases in the EDs, but the appropriate disposition and discharge of these patients may take days or even weeks. Visiting a busy ED with five to seven patients waiting for psychiatric beds is not unusual. This is further confounded by the number of psychiatric emergencies complicated by underlying significant medical conditions. There are also many individuals in the older age groups where dementia and similar illnesses may complicate placement. The number of available psychiatric beds is small, and even less available are the number of med-psych or geriatric-psych beds in even large communities.

4.   Homelessness

✓ Somewhere between one-third and one-half of homeless patients seeking medical care have drug/alcohol or significant psychiatric illness complicating their social issues. The crisis that we now see has been adjudicated by some communities that have actively enlarged or developed homeless facilities. This has been accomplished by attenuating existing prohibitions on the development of mini-houses and by expanding state and federal medical coverage of the expanding homeless population. There has also been a considerable impact on local and community charitable support groups providing meals and showers. Communities have collaborated in committing space and personnel at schools and colleges, for example, to care for homeless patients during the pandemic.

✓ The causes of homelessness are multiple, but the bottom line is that the safety net for this population is the emergency department. The ED is already impacted by community-wide limitations of access to nonemergent medical services, the frequent holes in the financial safety net, and the competition for beds by Covid patients. The long-term impact of the Covid pandemic and its consequent demand for services has impacted the homeless situation and will even more as we look toward the future.

✗ In the emergency department and the acute care hospital setting, these social determinants of health occupy tremendous resources. Their impact on the staff is also intense, both short-term at the bedside and even more so in terms of job satisfaction and burnout. These patients make the necessary emotional commitment and connection with our patients much more complex. It is a credit to the care providers for their continued excellent services under the most challenging circumstances.

Our personal and systemic biases may also impact the patients within the categories above. One of the CMO (chief medical officers), Dr. George Collins, from a hospital where I worked, was called to get involved with a patient in the intensive care unit. Despite being in critical shape, the patient was verbally abusing the staff. The patient was homeless and had a significant history of alcohol and drug use. The team wanted to know if they could just let the patient go, call the police, or chemically sedate him. None of these solutions was ideal, so rather than "approve one," the CMO went immediately in person to the ICU.

In his mind, patient safety was primary, but so was the safety of the clinical staff. To be protected against Covid or other infectious diseases was paramount, but so was preventing bodily or emotional harm to the treating team. This patient had a history of hitting caregivers, and the staff was quite wary of him and his behaviors.

Dr. Collins approached this difficult patient warily. After several confrontational starts, he ascertained that the patient wanted to leave the hospital because he had his dog parked on a public street in his motor home. Many patients in all social categories prioritize the care of their animals over themselves. The patient's motor home would not start. Dr. Collins was not deterred and with considerable effort and planning was able to have it moved to the hospital parking lot.

The CMO and other staff members then volunteered to take turns walking the patient's dog and being sure there was adequate food and water. The patient completed his hospital stay and lived in his motor home on hospital property for some time, supervised by the CMO and staff, who also chipped in to repair his motor home. (This is one of those "don't ask, don't tell" stories.)

Communication between the caregiving team and the patient was possible by stepping out of the confrontational *bias* created on both sides and, fortunately, enabled a positive outcome. This is not to say that the positive bias about the patient's dog didn't also play an essential role in this story.

✈ Bias is an ongoing fact in all aspects of life. Kahneman and Tversky, in multiple papers and books, [(70), (71), (72)] demonstrated bias in economic and mathematical decision-making. In his books on emotional intelligence, Goleman also deals with bias on a gut level. Our goal, when dealing with individual patients, or on a much larger level dealing with massive data (the third **WHAT**), is to recognize that our biases exist, understand them, and be able to deal with them situationally to minimize the impact on our interpretations and our decision making.

✦ One of the other difficulties that these populations, impacted by the social determinants of disease, provoke is understanding how these patients impact the system's national data sets. The scope of the problem of alcohol/drug use, psychiatric issues, and homelessness, either independently or mashed together as they frequently are, confounds the understanding of both process and outcome data. As a significant factor in understanding the baseline of all our quality measures, these populations as well as Covid patients make the national health- care data much more difficult to understand.

Several software programs are now available to help prioritize the care of complex or complicated patients, including the impact of psycho-social and drug issues. Identifying these problems at the time of care rather than at the time of discharge is a valuable upgrade. When integrated with the facility's mainframe capacity, these programs can also project patient needs and add significantly to the efforts to provide continuity and post-acute care.

✦ *Readmissions* to the acute care hospital and revisits to an emergency department have become significant markers for the quality of care. As with the patient Max Halter, described in the last few pages, Max illustrates two sets of data that hugely impact hospitals, health care systems, and national quality reporting. Inpatient length of stay and readmissions have far-reaching implications.

The limitations of process data in representing the gold standard of quality and the lack of timeliness and focus of outcome data are significant challenges in utilizing this incredibly valuable information. When presented with the firehouse gush of data, at least monthly and even daily in some situations, we are challenged to "choose wisely," as the knight from the movie *Indiana Jones and the Last Crusade* told Indy.

There are many competing forces for the resources necessary to effectively compile data, validate it, prioritize it, and then actually use the data to improve care. One of the most disadvantageous approaches is reacting to the "grade" from an agency or evaluating group. It is not uncommon for the refrain at the executive or corporate level to be "What do we need to do to get from a B to an A?" Unfortunately, this tends to focus on the mathematics of grade achievement rather than on the rich opportunities for improvement that the data presents.

Many quality and safety teams use a cascade approach to look at the *extensive* amount of data sets available, locally, geographically, and nationally. The third **W** is a consolidation of the first elements of the cascade data, validation, and prioritization. The fourth **W** is analysis, and the fifth **W** is education and, most importantly, *doing something*.

There are many data sources available with an increasingly successful methodology for collection. Initially, data was collected through actual observation of patient care. Those old enough will remember clipboards in the hands of administrative associates checking off items, times, and fulfillment of standards. This methodology was directed at better understanding the various processes that constituted a specific care pattern. Very time- and resource-intensive, this data collection was often left in the hands of various outside consultants.

After the laborious collation of data, there was often a report suggesting a positive change to various aspects of care before the departure of the consultants. This approach depended on the theory that "if we show them, they will change." The choice of studied items was often obscure and frequently did not try to answer critical questions but rather only provoke improvements simply by change itself. Initially, we measured what we could, collecting easily retrievable data rather than trying to answer the most pressing issues.

Quality analytics started with an experienced nurse, Betty Frask (whom we met earlier), spending hundreds of hours manually reviewing charts. I can remember her office well. Piles of patient charts shadowed the light from her window. There was never an endpoint in the number of hours she dedicated to extracting information from the clinical records that later were summarized and became critical data sets. This data became the basis for essential meetings and conversations in developing *process improvement* activities. To her credit, she captured the essence of care and tabulated it to some degree. She was highly experienced and motivated and facilitated the push to take information and use it to produce knowledge, which, as T. S. Eliot said, could lead to *wisdom*.

As time went on, Betty incorporated standards and compliance guidelines that became increasingly available from specialty societies and TJC (The Joint Commission on Hospital Standards). These elements became a quality and safety grid that, through education and some punitive measures, further forced hospitals to perform in a quality fashion without significant deviation from the increasing body of well-accepted standards.

The next battle came from the "naysayers" who questioned the validity of the data, mainly as it was used compared to data streams from divergent situations. Although there was recognition of discrepancies, as *statistical models* became more prevalent, the data carried more and more of a truthful and significant message.

Validation today is one of the absolutely essential elements of the data cascade, ultimately moving in the direction of aggressively pointing toward improvement.

With the onset of computer-based record-keeping systems EHR (electronic health record), the consultants' clipboards were replaced with accumulating the most easily measured data. From the clinical practitioner standpoint, this increasing focus on numerically, almost overwhelming, data streams significantly undermined the clinical focus. The result was an increased *documentation* workload, which decreased the physician's time to contact the patients directly.

It was often argued that the data accumulation really had little impact compared with the seasoned practitioner's knowledge and experience. The complexity, variability, and uncertainty of patient care defied the electronic health record's standardized model. Sitting in staff meetings, even the elite clinical practitioners objected to the intrusion into their world by the demands of the EHR. Not only was the data suspect, but the safety measures inherent in the electronic record seemed to alter the patient focus further. Utilizing the electronic health record for documentation and computerized order entry for patient orders also commanded significantly more time and further diluted providers' energy at the bedside.

Statistical modeling of large data sets has somewhat defeated the objections heard loudly from physicians, but the argument (discussion) rages on in many quarters.

CODING

Further advances in electronic record-keeping have continued to refine the data stream. Betty Frank (our quality analyst) now only selectively reviews actual paper or computer-based records. Most of the outcome and even much of the process data is now based on codes.

Coding is a complex process that has also gone through a significant change. Initially, coders, who went through considerable education, training, and certification, reviewed medical records through the electronic health record. These professional coders assigned codes to diagnosis and treatments when a patient was hospitalized on the basis of definite rules and standards. Codes then became the basis of our data, particularly at the national level. Initially, codes were designed to facilitate finances and billing for the substantive diagnosis and procedures documented in the medical record. Government and private insurance companies pay based on codes when paying for care. It was much more efficient, controlled resources, and provided consistency. It also became the basis for data collection.

Originally, coders were part of the organization or hospital where the patients they were coding were seen. The coders knew the staff and the operational issues and could ask questions if necessary. Most recently, the coders mainly work for contract agencies and don't know the staff or the hospital providing services. *The government or insurance companies that pay the bills never see a patient and hardly ever see a paper or computerized record of patient care, only the codes.*

The coding/billing/data process is further complicated by the CAC (computer-assisted coding). There are multiple variations on this theme, but basically, it is an artificial intelligence system that relies heavily on word recognition. The coding done by CAC is "reviewed" by a certified coder, which should give additional credibility to the data derived from codes. It should be understood that the primary motivation for coding is financial and that CAC is used to increase the efficiency and standardization of coding. A contract coder, who is commonly working from home, may have multiple motivations. Having worked with many of these folks, they are highly focused and understand the importance of what they do, particularly as it impacts billing and compliance. However, pressures on productivity play an important role in the incentives of the coder and can introduce the prioritization of time in the coding process itself.

4. Sometimes lost in the complexity of the coding process is the downstream importance in terms of how the codes impact the data on diagnosis and care. As structured, this process requires significant oversight and can significantly impact the data and all the downstream reporting that relies on it. Codes may seriously impact quality goals, program incentives for facilities, management and leadership, national grades, and government incentives and penalties. Many of the coders I initially talked to had no idea of their impact on a given facility's quality and rating process. This was particularly true with "offshore" coders employed by some agencies. Much like the common usage of IT support personnel, offshore coders are often from India and the Philippines. These individuals commonly did not have the experience or educational opportunities in medical coding afforded to our best homegrown contractors.

We spent significant time in weekly meetings with our contract coders and their leadership. As with many of the themes in this book, the elements of developing a compatible, high-functioning process depend on the commitment and accountability of the individuals involved. A dedicated, focused meeting of the involved individuals was dynamic, problem-solving in nature, educational, and necessary to have a" gut-level" or midbrain attachment to the end product. In this case, the sum of all the parts and actions was only superficially coded, but the details were actually necessary to impact a patient's care and life.

The translation of the complex medical record is impacted by more than just the coder's expertise. They must focus on more than the primary diagnosis, and there is a strict limitation on how much time they can spend in the process. There are significant concerns about the validity of computer-assisted coding, and even about the stated priority of the ultimate coding goal.

Underlying all these aspects is the quality of documentation by the clinical team. The coders will tell you, "If it's not documented, it can't be coded." Although the previous paragraphs focused on coding, the crux of the matter does sit with *documentation*.

The integration of the electronic health record had promised to address several issues in addition to the safety and redundancy elements discussed previously.

- Improved communication between multiple involved clinical elements. The primary physician has access, for example, to multiple team members' notes. This includes physical therapy, pharmacy, care coordination, social work, and nursing. Specialists seeing the patient had their notes immediately integrated into the electronic health record for all care providers to visualize. This became even more essential as much of the care of inpatients fell into the hands of hospitalists, who worked shifts and participated in many hand-offs to their colleagues.

- Increasing availability of current data and documented reports from various locations. A physician, for example, might visualize a test result on his patient from his office and have the ability to write orders and notes from offsite.

- Improved availability of hospital records to the patients themselves.

- Improved collaboration between hospitals and systems, extending beyond the traditional geographic catchment area.

For this scheme to work effectively, the comprehensiveness of the notes in the EHR had to improve, requiring more time and effort. Many systems have been developed to assist this documentation process. This included typing directly into any immediately available workstation, dictating notes to various immediate transcription services, and computer programs concurrently translating the spoken to written words immediately. In some situations, "scribe" assistants have been utilized to record dictation, observe and document an exam, integrate diagnostic studies, and record patient questions and instructions.

Of late, there are also examples of "Google Glasses" that a caregiver can utilize to do *much of what an onboard scribe can accomplish.* Alex Web reported in Big Techs New Vision (73) that the current Glasses now available are only early steps by Big Tech to engineer reality and virtual reality in the immediate vision of folks from gamers to professionals.

The caregiver must then spend significant time with the "machine," which unfortunately takes away from time directly with the patient. When physicians were forced to convert to the EHR (Electronic Health Record) from the paper record, there was an immediate drop of approximately 30 percent in the capacity of physicians to see patients in the acute hospital setting. Some of this has been recouped as caregivers have learned the science of the electronic health record, but not all. In addition, the computer has become a physical and psychological barrier between the caregiver and the patient. When one makes rounds in an acute care hospital, most staff are at their workstations, not with the patients. This is true for the nursing and support staff, even though they have formidable bedside tasks.

There have however been multiple enhancements to the primary electronic health record on the compliance side *to increase efficiency*. One of these changes is the ability and allowance that daily physician notes may be literally copied and pasted into the next day, with "updates." This theory is that information can be brought forward and added to without rewriting an entire note. This, of course, is a tremendous time saver. However, in the busy life of the caregiver, it is easier to copy and paste, filling the chart with duplicative, redundant, and somewhat confusing verbiage. This frequently is a significant disadvantage for other caregivers or support staff trying to make sense of a patient's progress.

The art of physician documentation, for communication, coding, and quality review, and even for legal purposes, continues to be problematic. Therefore, coders, even the excellent ones, cannot truly reflect the patient's care. A new industry in this field has grown to support this process. Teams of experts comb the patient charts while still in the hospital. On the basis of the existing diagnostics and therapies, they will query caregivers, without prompting them, to add further documentation in diagnosis and explanations of care.

Quality and safety teams at the hospitals have added their own expert coders to review charts that need documentation improvement, particularly in focus areas such as sepsis, readmissions, and patient safety issues. Compliance in these areas is rigorously adhered to. There is no leading a physician to documentation that doesn't reflect absolute care. Instead, it presents the coding process as an opportunity to reflect on the actual care and the documentation of what the patient received.

The need for all of these options for documentation is multiplied as approaches to care such as "telehealth," distal at-home monitoring, and patient portals increasingly become the fundamental elements of health care.

The actual end product in medicine or many other fields is much more difficult to ascertain. To some executives, an A grade, or 5-star rating, or whatever the marker, is the most positive reflection of the end product. Although easy to publicize, the grade is not what leadership or culture is about. An A grade is nice to have but cannot replace the belief that the publicized numerical or letter grade is not the endpoint as a team member. It only represents a step in raising the standard of care for patients and the standard of care for a specific patient.

✗ The next evolution in data collection, at the local, system, and national levels, is the direct scanning of charts electronically. This addition to the current coding process would seem to be a positive response to some of the deficits of the current accuracy of codes. Although undoubtedly true, the exclusion of Betty Frask and those with her skills, the other quality people she represents, and the contract coders, eliminate the human quality review they provide.

Next, we must understand the various data sources, how they are derived, and the best mechanism for validation. Process and outcome data must be dissected before resources are committed, and vast amounts of energy are spent responding. We innocently asked for more data to assist in the process improvement activities. We now have hundreds of data points that need to be evaluated. A selection methodology helps in resource allocation in the quality data cascade, with multiple data sets, multiple indexes, and widely variable reporting models.

To prevent drowning in data, we have used an **IOI** (**Intuitive Opportunity Index**), which helps to break down significant data sets into attributes. An example of the utilization of the IOI shows why some of the high-priority data measures are selected for prioritization.

MEASURE	Process vs Outcome	Proximity to goal	Appearance on matrices	$ impact	Direct pt. impact	Potential impact on data	Point total
Death from pneumonia	30 points	20	20	0	20	10	100 pts
7–30-day readmissions	30 points	20	10	30	30	20	140

C-diff infections	30	10	20	10	30	10	110
Sepsis bundle compliance	20	10	10	20	30	10	100
Efficient radiology	10	30	10	20	10	30	110
Two-day observation compliance	20	0	10	20	0	10	60

The IOI is a simple scoring system that evaluates data sets for their strength and relevance to the multiple attributes of care. The details are then each scored on a 10-20-30 point scale.

The attributes are as follows:

1. How many patients are impacted?

   a. Is the event a very rare statistical occurrence (a significant safety issue)?

   b. It is important to know the numerator and denominator of a measure. For example, the number of eligible patients who receive prophylaxis to prevent clotting after an elective knee or hip surgery relative to those that do not.

2. How often does this factor, process, and outcome apply?

   a. Is this data reflective of a frequent occurrence in the care of patients, such as the timing of an EKG in a patient with chest pain presenting to the ED (high frequency)?

3. Is the data stream timely and how timely?

a. Process data can be looked at daily or even every hour in some circumstances. CMS (Center for Medicare Services, government) data has been running for one to three years old. In addition, it is often presented as cumulative data over a three-year time frame.

4. Can the data or information actually impact the care of the patient at the time the care is being delivered? For example, knowing that a core neonatal blood test to rule out jaundice at the time a baby is still at risk in the hospital can be life-saving.

5. Does the process measure impact resource utilization and the timing of care?

6. Does the data impact finance directly? Some measurable processes are in place to ensure that resource utilization and costs are appropriate. In addition, some process and outcome measures have direct government and insurer incentives and disincentives that can be seriously impactful.

7. Does the data come from programs with the possibility of incentives or disincentives?

8. How does this data impact bottom-line finance?

    a. Some governmental data impacts multiple programs as either incentives or disincentives.

9. Does the data impact ratings and grades?

10. How far away is the data from the goal?

    a. Should resource be put toward data that is quite far from the goal?

    b. Should resources be put toward data improvement that is close but not entirely at goal?

11. How difficult is the remedy, and how much will it cost financially and resource utilization?

12. How much impact does this data feature have on other related aspects of care? (For example, how does the arrival time for EKG significantly impact the time it takes a patient with an acute MI to get to the Cath lab?

13. How long has this data set been an issue?

14. On how many national scorecards does this data set appear?

15. How much does this one data set impact the overall rating of a hospital, clinic, or system?

16. How much do people inside and outside the industry really care about this?

17. Are, or can there be, resources available to impact a significant change?

It should be noted that the process is defined as an *intuitive* opportunity index because the ultimate selection of opportunities is guided initially by the scoring system. Still, the human element, EI, and intuition are also factored in. The people delivering care weigh in and can fundamentally impact a more comprehensive assessment than available with only the scoring system. This can also significantly impact when we talk about the fifth **W** in our model (**What** can we do about it).

There are as many as six hundred data points per month available for review, hence the description earlier of drinking from a firehouse. Once a few data sets are highlighted, prioritized, and validated, the real work begins. For example, the several data streams below will illustrate the utilization of the Intuitive Opportunity Index and look more carefully at the distinction between outcome and process measures.

- **Length of Stay:** This is an outcome measure reflecting the efficiency and cost of care.

- **Severe sepsis:** The data from the overall care of sepsis patients combines information from process measures and national outcome data.

- **Readmissions:** The overall percentage of 30-day readmissions, of five selected diagnostic categories, is powerful outcome data.

- **Mortality** This "gold standard "outcome data is only available from CMS

- **Efficient use of radiology** (with and without contrast material process data) is a process measure.

Of the copious mountains of data now available, the intuitive opportunity index has helped us select the five issues bulleted above, as an example, for focus and action. LOS, severe sepsis, readmission, mortality, and efficient use of radiology all made the cut on the basis of the IOI results. Without going into actual hospital data, the first four items were conspicuous for their importance, visibility, impact on patients, availability of concurrent or very recent data, and immediate impact on patient care. One of the intuitive opportunity index considerations was embracing those data sets that realistically, with existing resources, could be immediately impacted.

It should be noted that the government mainly has become increasingly adept at providing information in a much timelier fashion and scorecards that help providers understand their focus. Working closely with several external and internal agencies has allowed us to develop internal scorecards that *project opportunities* even from preliminary data. That has become a serious factor as we try to index our priorities. For example, waiting for data from the government, which may be as many as three years old, for the death rate in patients hospitalized with pneumonia has limited value. Projecting a trend for the last three to six months realistically allows for in-depth evaluations of the course of these patients. This also provides an opportunity to study the issues and initiate process improvement immediately. Knowing in advance, or even currently, the most pressing opportunities allow the team to develop an aggressive short-term plan and a longer-term strategy.

A *matrix approach* also helps everyone to be on the same page. The data is shared with the entire organization. The whole operational team can then develop a fundamental understanding and trust in the data. This is different from a "show and tell" at a board meeting, executive level, or staff meeting. The distribution literally goes to everyone. It is not someone else's data, but it is closely approximated to their work and becomes their own.

Ownership of the data is critical because focusing solely on **WHAT** (the data) is only an initial step and the hard work of understanding the **WHY**. It requires input from the people who provide day-to-day and moment-to-moment care. This is the difference maker! This analysis must be done not only in the teams who live primarily in the data but also by people who do the work and understand the consequences of their work. The data becomes the substrate for team meetings that favor ownership, accountability, and personal involvement. This is the data for "my patient."

EFFICIENT USE OF RADIOLOGY

✶ Considering the IOI, why would the efficient use of radiology be chosen relative to the other more significant items? Did it impact patient care in the same way as the more apparent selections? Efficient use of radiology has been measured by high-end radiologic procedures, such as CT scans and MRI, performed *with and without contrast material.* Contrast is given intravenously or orally, highlighting certain exam features. Government auditors are looking at this seemingly mathematical data set with great interest. It represents the potential for doing unnecessary exams that double the cost and, more importantly, put the patients at risk for unwanted exposure. The average percentage of these exams, with and without contrast, nationally is usually just on the upside of 6 percent.

✶ When selecting other data sets to analyze, utilizing the IOI (intuitive opportunity index), this does not seem to be a prominent place for time or resources. When looking at all the national matrices, in comparison, this data set seemed very insignificant, that is until examined critically, which pointed to a very high percentage of these exams, as much as 26 percent at a single facility. The rate of radiological studies with and without contrast was so significantly above the national average that this one data set had an untoward effect on the total point collection and, therefore, a substantial downward drag on the total score on CMS star ratings. It effectively gave an excellent hospital a 3- or 4-star rating instead of a 5-star rating, which most of the other metrics would have warranted.

LENGTH OF STAY (LOS)

Beth Calder, a fifty-two-year-old patient with a history of CLL (chronic lymphocytic leukemia), was admitted to the hospital with a cough and fever. A chest X-ray revealed that she had right lower lobe pneumonia in the emergency department. One week before, she had taken care of her seven-year-old grandchild, who had an upper respiratory infection. The diagnosis in the ED was pneumonia, and the patient was admitted for IV antibiotics. Most patients in her age group might have been started on oral antibiotics and sent home for careful follow-up, but she was admitted because of her underlying leukemia.

Beth was not actively receiving cancer therapy for her lymphocytic leukemia. After three days in the hospital, she was afebrile, eating and drinking well, and moving about the hospital towing her IV pole and antibiotics.

⚹ The care of all hospitalized patients now includes a *care coordinator* (sometimes called a *case manager* in some hospital systems). The coordinator's role provides discharge planning, integrates multiple disciplines, and ensures patients can be appropriately and safely discharged. This role includes knowing the GMLOS (Geometric Length of Stay) for Beth's diagnosis and planning for compliance with that indicator. The GMLOS is the geometric length of stay, which is quite diagnosis-specific and is assigned by the government on the basis of massive national average data sets. It is a very significant factor in calculating the payment of a patient's care.

✓ Before the current milieu, payment for hospitalization was based on time and materials, as in how many days the patient was in the hospital and what was used and what was done, such as IV antibiotics, tests, and other procedures.

✱ Currently, the government and most insurers pay contracted rates based on the patient's DRG (Diagnostic Related Group). Beth would fall into "uncomplicated pneumonia, with stable CLL." This would have a GMLOS of 3.5 days, and no matter how long she stayed in the hospital and, for the most part, what was done while she was there, the bill for her care would be paid based on the GMLOS.

✱ Most contracted payments barely meet the *cost* of care if the LOS is rigidly adhered to. It is now generally understood that the most appropriate time for discharge from the hospital is when the patient is *better*. Delaying the release until the patient is *well* is not realistic. Several reasons demand and facilitate this protocol:

✱ • Finance: Payors no longer pay for services, such as room day rates, nursing care, medications, support services, etc. Utilizing the governmental model of DRG payments, the reimbursement received by the hospital is based roughly on a DRG payment schedule. These are calculated on a cost basis relative to the diagnosis. A patient with pneumonia, for example, receives a payment based on an ALOS (average length of stay) for a diagnosis coded as uncomplicated pneumonia). It is not to anyone's *financial advantage*, either the hospital, government, insurance company, or even the patient, to remain in the hospital.

• ✓ Safety: Hospitals are not inherently safe places. As we have seen most dramatically with Covid, the multiplicity of patients in the inpatient setting is an opportunity for disease transference. In addition, multiplying the number of things that happen to patients each day, medications, tests, procedures, food, movement, bath rooming, and many others, as well as the number of patients coming in and out, increases the probabilities of "bad things" happening.

- ✓ Resource utilization: We have seen circumstantially that there are fixed resources available for medical services. Factors such as the seasonal flu and pandemics can step well beyond available resources. The vivid pictures of the large hospitals in New York City overwhelmed by patients during the initial Covid siege are memories none of us will ever forget.

- ✗ Business model: Medical care more and more functions along with a business model. Inpatient hospital services make up a significant cost of care. Getting patients out helps to keep the model alive.

- ✗ Alternative care: There has been a significant increase in post-acute availability that allows for earlier discharges from the hospital. Over a week or two, rehab units facilitate the return of hospitalized patients to normalcy. Home health allows for continued care, observation, and treatment of patients in their natural home setting. Home-monitoring capabilities are growing nationally that allow for technology to be brought post-discharge into the home, facilitating the care of patients, particularly those with chronic illnesses.

- ✗ Care coordination (case management): Many inpatient facilities and systems now take responsibility for coordinating the care of patients *across the continuum.* Everything from follow-up problem-saving phone calls after discharge, following patients at all levels of care, and facilitating coordination and communication of a team approach in and outside the hospital setting helps soften the significant downgrading of care when a patient leaves the hospital. Remember, for the most part, patients are better, not well, when discharged.

- In Beth's case, her hospitalization and its cost were complicated by her hematologist, who was consulted on the case and ordered some more specialized testing to evaluate the status of her underlying leukemia better. The care coordinator on the case called the hematologist and informed him that the testing could be done as an outpatient. Still, the physician insisted that the tests be done before discharge since it was much easier for the patient than having her return to the hospital for further testing.

The consequences of Beth staying in the hospital two more days over her GMLOS with a length of stay of 5.5 days were as follows:

- The inability of the hospital to receive payment for the cost of additional care.

- Depending on the insurer, since Medicare did not cover Beth, the patient might have to assume a significant portion of the cost of additional inpatient days and testing

- Beth, with weakened immunity, was potentially exposed to multiple other contagious disease processes (This is despite meticulous hospital-wide cleaning, sterilization, and infection prevention methodology.).

- Decreased bed availability for other sicker patients, particularly during a pandemic like Covid or even a seasonal epidemic like the flu.

- A suggestion in the data on some national and system dashboards that the facility was not managing its processes efficiently and effectively and the consequent penalties that might be associated.

The focus on the role of care coordination in these hospitalized circumstances should not undermine the understanding of the importance of their role in *care coordination across the continuum*. Often referred to as discharge planners, one of the primary functions of care coordination is financial. They must communicate and coordinate the complex contractual relationships that characterize inpatient hospitalizations.

In the face of the current state of health care, the care coordinator's role is incredibly impactful in managing post-acute patterns, particularly in patients where social determinants play a significant role. For example, Medicare does not cover long-term health facilities unless the patient meets specific nursing or medical services requirements. Finding a facility that can care for a Medicare-qualified older patient without long-term health insurance is often a daunting problem.

The hospital must ensure that a patient has a *safe discharge*. In California, Senate Bill 675 became effective January 2016, requiring hospitals to arrange for appropriate post-hospital care. For Medicare patients and their family caregivers, the law increases the opportunity to participate in the discharge process. Every patient, including those with no resources, must have a place to go, appropriate clothing, and access to medical and supportive services. Most communities face severe resource issues during the post-acute phase of care.

SNFS (Skilled nursing facilities) are licensed to care for very specific types of patients; for example, they cannot treat patients with primary psychiatric or behavioral issues. As institutions, SNFs only take patients with some funding sources. Patients with social determinants of disease take up a disproportionate amount of time in providing continuity of care and adhering to the letter of SB 675. Home Health also has specific limitations as to which patients qualify for their services. Although Medicare and other insurers will cover qualified Home Health visits, a significant number are funded by the discharging hospital to provide this service, which has financial consequences but is a significant advantage in preventing hospital readmissions and enhancing continuity.

Follow-up appointments with a care provider are frequently problematic, even in patients with a private physician. Patients released from the hospital that do not have an appointment with a doctor within two weeks are significantly more likely to need either rehospitalization or acute level care, such as in the emergency department. Data from HSAG (the Health Services Advisory Group), which is the Quality Innovation Network (QIN)-Quality Improvement Organization (QIO) for California and Arizona, report an almost 50 percent increase in readmissions in those patients without follow-up

✓ care within two weeks after hospital discharge. As the continuity of care of patients has deteriorated for multiple reasons, the care coordinator's job has become much more complex, which sometimes makes compliance with GMLOS problematic.

Length of stay can be interpreted as an outcome measure but is measured chiefly as a series of process measures. It is also heavily impacted by local medical services and the health of the local social services network. This includes homeless shelters and programs, the availability of acute and chronic psychiatric services, and the penetration of community alcohol and drug programs. As is reasonable to expect, the above issues also significantly impact the readmission probability of patients discharged from the acute care setting.

READMISSIONS

In a certain sense, readmissions and length of stay represent the yin and yang of hospitalized patients. Common sense might indicate an inverse relationship between keeping patients in the hospital longer and the probability of readmission. First, let's understand the rules: A readmission must be considered unnecessary in this statistic. That means that patients brought back to the hospital after a qualifying stay on an elective basis are not included in this group. Patients that are returned, for example, for elective procedures or elective surgery or additional scheduled intravenous chemotherapy are not in the numerator of this equation.

⤳ Readmissions get very high scores on the intuitive opportunity index for several reasons.

↧ The data appears on multiple local and national scorecards.

- The composite data is relatively available in a short time frame and, therefore, can lead to process improvement.

- There are EHR platforms that focus on alerts and coordination that can lead to immediate direct individual patient care improvements.

- Readmission data is tiered, recognizing the importance of social determinants of disease.

- Readmissions cost providers and payors significant dollars.

- * The government has integrated significant penalties for readmissions (acute MI, COPD, pneumonia, hip and knee replacements). Readmissions are one of three CMS programs that invoke penalties at this writing.

- Jason Mills was a sixty-seven-year-old male who finally elected to have hip replacement surgery. Six months prior, he finally was referred to an orthopedist because of increasing pain in his left hip and limping even on short walks. The original evaluation included radiological studies that demonstrated "bone on bone," and the specialist recommended hip replacement therapy. "How do I know when it is time to have this surgery?" Jason asked his doctor, only to be told that "he would know," meaning that the pain and disability would worsen until he couldn't take it anymore.

Jason's orthopedist wasn't surprised when he got the call five months later, and he started the presurgical process for hip replacement.

Jason had an uncomplicated surgical course, and after two nights in the hospital, demonstrating safe ambulation and an appropriate home care situation, he was discharged. It should be noted, as of this writing, that many new techniques have been developed that have significantly impacted the expected length of stay of patients like Jason, and orthopedic replacement procedures have been converted to outpatient with patients going home the same day as surgery.

After two weeks at home, Jason's boredom got the best of him, and shunning his walker for a cane, he left his home with the intention of a short neighborhood walk. He did not appreciate the speed of a car coming his way while crossing the street, and when he jumped back to avoid being hit, he fell and tried to spare his newly repaired hip. He fractured the ankle on his right leg. He was taken to the emergency department and found to need immediate emergency surgery to stabilize and repair his injury. Since he was readmitted within thirty days after his previous hip surgery, this hospital visit fell within the guidelines and was counted as a readmission. This was directly unrelated to his hip surgery, as is the case in many other "unnecessary readmissions," which have been the subject of much debate.

The government has made readmissions one of its three financial penalty programs. If a hospital generates above-expected data, the penalties can run into millions of dollars. Over the last several years, the government has become more sensitive to social determinants of disease and has responded with a tiered structure for readmission penalties. The system is based on five tiers. The government uses the percentage of Medicaid/Medicare patients to reflect the number of issues in patients where social issues confound their care. Particularly in recently discharged patients, this tiered system has significantly altered the thresholds of penalties and the financial penalties inflicted. Hospitals that deliver care to large numbers of patients with concurrent social issues have allowable higher limits to their readmission rates before governmental penalties.

State and Federal government programs utilize a thirty-day window for patient readmissions. Despite some of the previously mentioned problems, the readmission data represents a great *laboratory* to dissect the current issues impacting quality patient care. It is also a reflection on the disruption of *continuity* that has befallen our system and an opportunity to rebuild in a different model.

The thirty-day readmission mark is available through CMS as a national comparison and at the state level by hospital and region and is a valuable comparison as a benchmark. Many of the patients in this category have long-term chronic diseases such as heart failure and chronic obstructive lung disease. Most hospital systems have designed and implemented resources to address these patients. One of the most important is recognizing end-stage disease management and the critical need for "goals of care" conversations. A palliative care program is the heart and soul of discussions empowering patients to take charge of their last six months of life in many hospital systems.

More recently, individual hospitals and systems are utilizing a seven-day benchmark. This seven-day readmission data reveals significant other opportunities. It is more focused on what issues are apparent.

- Care coordination across the continuum

- Discharge planning

- Medication availability

- Transportation

- Post-discharge phone calls

- Discharge instructions

- Home Health

- Post-discharge placement

- Social determinants

- Appropriate inpatient care before discharge

Brian Wilcox was a fifty-seven-year-old patient presenting to the ED with shaking, chills, and cough for several weeks. Paramedics found Brian in his car when a passerby noted him to be passed out in the back seat. Brian had become a feature in the neighborhood because his vehicle was constantly parked and moved only several blocks from one side of the street to another. It looked to the passerby to be full of filthy boxes and personal items. The local police department had been called to do "safety checks," and he had been referred to the homeless shelter without much compliance. He was diagnosed with severe sepsis in the ED and vigorously treated with antibiotics and fluids.

After an eight-day hospital course, Brian was up and around and was adamant about returning to his car, refusing any other, even short-term, placement. He could not get his prescriptions filled because of his social issues and was therefore dispensed medications from the hospital pharmacy. He was given an appointment to see a clinic doctor for a follow-up in five days, which he promised to keep and was given a cab voucher to assist in keeping his scheduled visit.

Brian did not show up for his visit, and despite multiple calls to the number he provided the care management staff, he could not be reached. Four days later, he was readmitted to the hospital after paramedics once again brought him to the emergency department since he was found unconscious in his car.

✦ Patients presenting with a primary diagnosis of severe sepsis on their initial hospital visit have over a 30 percent *readmission rate*, predominantly with sepsis again within thirty days. Forty percent of these patients readmit within the first week after discharge, and 25 percent readmit within seventy-two hours. When considering where to dedicate scarce hospital resources, readmissions, especially those for sepsis, seem to be a good bet.

Similar data within other major diagnostic groups are available and serve as an excellent laboratory for evaluating the total care of our patients across the continuum. Unfortunately, Brian represents a challenging group of patients. Still, some of the issues presented in his case are part of the fundamental disruption of the continuity of care in our current health care model.

A couple of years ago, readmission data was directed at the rebound phenomenon of patients enrolled in a compliance-qualifying inpatient setting and was counted only when they returned to a similar inpatient setting. After a "trial" period, the government has put EDAC (Excess Days In Acute Care) into hospital performance standards. These EDAC standards represent the effort to corral unnecessary clinical intervention in addition to the classical inpatient readmission. EDAC gives points (½ point) for a revisit to the emergency department or readmission to an observation bed (this was not previously counted). Some facilities had used the latter to reduce penalties from regular readmissions. In addition, as opposed to inpatient readmission being counted as one, the number of readmission days is also calculated. As of this writing, the EDAC measures for this year have not yet been tabulated.

Readmission is only one of three programs used by the government to judge quality and safety. These programs are used to inflict *penalties* or reward incentives to hospitals. Two of these programs, including readmissions, are penalty programs only. The other penalty-only program is *patient safety events*. Depending again on national outcome performance, the government penalizes complications (including deaths) in patients receiving hospital-level care from very specific areas:

- Acute myocardial infarction (heart attack)

- Pneumonia

- Congestive heart failure

- Chronic obstructive lung disease (COPD)

- Knee and hip replacements

- Post GI surgery

The third program is **VBP** (value-based purchasing). This program has a financial impact based on the redistribution of dollars through penalties to a small (approximately 10 percent) of hospitals that competitively have achieved the best results in the VBP program. The program's attractiveness comes from the fact that, if hospital scores at a competitive break-even, they get money equal to 2 percent "tine" on all operational payments taxed the previous year. This is reflected as a percentage increase in direct payments to hospitals for the following year. Bonus payments come from money deducted from those hospitals that do not achieve scores that trigger total or at least partial payments. The government does not have to put in their dollars but uses monies collected as taxes or penalties and doesn't redistribute that until the following calendar year.

Readmissions also have a big part in *patient satisfaction* and the resulting scores in many national quality/safety matrices. Patient satisfaction scores come from surveys filled out by patients and their families soon after discharge from the inpatient setting. This HCAPHS (Hospital Consumer Assessment of Healthcare Providers and Systems) survey consists of twenty-seven items and reflects recently discharged patients' opinions about the hospital experience. Communication with doctors and nurses, the responsiveness of hospital staff, and questions about cleanliness and quietness are scored. Similar surveys are now being used to evaluate ambulatory services such as emergency departments and clinics. These surveys are a conglomerate of questions with a rating scale.

The scores from the patient satisfaction surveys are assigned top box, middle box, and bottom box. Only top box scores of nine or ten out of ten are counted, reflecting positive answers. There is no credit unless one of the top two choices is selected. For example, how often discharge instructions were explained to you effectively. Hospitals strive to be in the 90th-plus percentile in all the HCAPHS survey questions.

Needing to return to the hospital, particularly in those patients that return in the first seven days, raises the concern that they were sent home too early. Many patients feel that they are not ready for discharge. The parameters have changed as mentioned; patients need to be *better* and do not have to continue for days in an acute care bed or even weeks until they are *well*.). This is a common dissatisfier and underscores the need for one-to-one communication and education as essential aspects of the transfer of patients to the next level of care (Note: The term "transfer" rather than "discharge" was used because leaving the hospital represents a tremendous transition for all patients, no matter what the diagnosis, and must be treated with the same comprehensiveness as if transferring a patient from the intensive care unit to the step-down unit.).

Severe Sepsis

✓ Apart from its readmission potential, the early recognition of severe sepsis, aggressive treatment, mortality rate, and adherence to standardized protocols also score highly on the IOI (intuitive opportunity index).

Thomas Conner was a seventy-six-year-old gentleman, trying not to slow down and deny the aging process, who had a long history of pretty well-controlled type II diabetes mellitus. Tom was well recognized in his neighborhood for his head of flowing grey hair and the fact that, rain or shine, he always wore shorts. Tom managed his illness with diet and oral medications without daily injections of insulin. He was quite active and prided himself that he played paddle ball at least three times per week with a group of men and women who were considerably younger than he was.

After a particularly energetic afternoon at the courts, he noted a blister on his left great toe. This, of course, was not the first time, so initially, he did not pay much attention to it. When he awoke the following day, he noted significant redness around the blister.

Blisters from his tennis shoes were not a new occurrence for Tom, and other than putting a Band-Aid on his lesion, he ignored it, although it was becoming increasingly uncomfortable. He didn't tell his wife because he thought she would scold him for not taking better care of himself. He limped into bed that evening, took acetaminophen for the discomfort, and covered the blister with a Band-Aid. He had a headache when he awoke the following morning after a fitful night.

His wife finally demanded to see his foot as he continued to limp around the house and not do

his weekly chores. After removing the dressing, she noted that the blistered area was red and very tender. She applied local topical antibiotic ointment, changed the dressing, and gave him a "serious what for" before she got into bed and turned off the lights.

He canceled an afternoon haircut appointment the following day because he had absolutely no energy, as he told his wife. He refused dinner because he had no appetite and wanted to go to bed that evening. He thought he was "coming down with something" and hoped a good night's sleep would help. His wife wanted him to at least call his doctor, but he refused and then again turned away from each other and put off the bedside tabletop lights.

At 4:00 a.m., his wife woke because of Tom's moaning, and she noted he was quite warm to touch and wasn't himself. She was worried it was his diabetes, and after trying to call his doctor without immediate success, she dialed 911.

On arrival at the ED, the patient was immediately put onto a gurney, where the ED team undressed him and noted that his pulse was rapid and that his blood pressure was low. They immediately started IV fluids, and after blood cultures and tests were sent to the laboratory, Tom was started on intravenous antibiotics.

The diagnosis of sepsis was confirmed, and the patient was admitted to the ICU (intensive care unit) for continued aggressive treatment. It was extremely fortunate that an intensive care unit bed was available for him, despite the significantly sustained influx of Covid-19 patients. The pandemic patients not only required the highest level of care and needed ventilators but remained in the ICU for weeks to even months rather than days.

Three harrowing days followed as the intensive care unit team supported Tom. At the same time, his immunity and high potency antibiotics fought the overwhelming infection. Days later, Tom, "as weak as a kitten," was transferred to the medical floor. After seven more days, he received physical therapy to regain his walking capabilities and was finally released from the hospital. "I never expected to be slammed as hard by anything. I knew I was sick, but I thought I was still in pretty good shape. All from a little blister," Tom exclaimed to his doctor. After several weeks of recovery, Tom could slowly return to his regular activities and finally, to the applause of his friends, returned to the paddle ball courts.

⚄ Thomas Conner is an excellent example of the effective treatment of a critical and often fatal illness. Analyzing his care process also produces data that can be considered a quality indicator. Approximately ten to fifteen years ago, as some of the most egregious medical data became more apparent, the mortality from severe sepsis was well into the high 30% range. It was understood that sepsis, or an overwhelming infection, is often found in patients with serious chronic diseases and compromised immunity. It was almost acceptable to have a sky-high mortality rate. However, as some studies became clear that early recognition and aggressive early therapy could significantly reduce mortality to less than 10 percent, a methodology workbook became a standard process guideline for care.

Standard procedures were established, and specific mortality goals were publicized. The treatment of sepsis then became a series of processes that could be measured in real-time and judged against nationally comparable outcome statistics.

Without question, caregivers were gleeful that their excellent work seriously impacted a significant cause of mortality. As time progressed and the leadership demanded further improvements, there seemed to follow a natural plateau. It was argued that lower and lower mortality goals were unrealistic in the high-risk patient population.

This is where **What2Why** changes the dialogue from merely reaching a numerical goal to carefully analyzing each case by clinicians and those directly involved in the patient's care. They start to ask questions differently and utilize the insights to continue to look for opportunities for improvements.

✔ Sepsis is an excellent laboratory to dissect how quality measures can be used to improve the care of our patients. These patients and their care can be looked at as a series of *measurable processes* and also as *outcome data* when looking at mortality and readmissions. For the most part, the process measurements focus on hospital-based measures such as Sepsis Bundle Compliance, and readmissions. Mortality data, from such things as Pneumonia and Acute Myocardial Infarction, fall within the realm of outcome data on national matrices. Some of the bundle measures are as follows:

1. How long was the patient in the emergency department before the patient was medically evaluated?

2. Was the sepsis triage screening form filled out?

3. Were appropriate levels of fluid administered within the acceptable time frame?

4. Did the patient receive antibiotics within the acceptable three-hour time frame?

5. Were appropriate blood cultures sent within the proscribed time frame?

6. Was a marker for sepsis sent and then repeated in the timely clinical reevaluation period?

Similar markers are also studied if an inpatient develops signs and symptoms of sepsis. Much like the example stated earlier in the book of using aspirin on arrival to the emergency department to measure quality cardiac care, these process measures in treating sepsis reflect the quality of care and its timeliness. We know directly from multiple research studies that compliance with a standardized treatment bundle positively impacts the care of sepsis patients.

It should also be noted that careful reevaluation of the process measures often leads to a rethinking of the actions themselves. For example, the amount of intravenous fluid in severe sepsis in the initial treatment time frame recommended has been in dispute for a long time. Most recently, there has been a serious reevaluation of the quantity of fluids, administration speed, and even the duration of fluids. This is not unexpected in medicine, where variability and uncertainty make large long-term data sets necessary and thoughtful evaluation mandatory. It is also why the government has not yet placed sepsis in a category that impacts financial incentives and penalties. There is still too much uncertainty in treating such a wide range of patients in almost innumerable circumstances.

It should be recognized that these and other specific process goals help in different ways and provide us with information on how we are doing. They focus attention and resources on specific patient populations and illnesses with significant care opportunities.

As with bundle compliance, process goals can help us standardize our approach to the complexities that present with complicated diagnoses such as sepsis. They parallel the computer-based and paper-based checklists that Atul Gawande has so eloquently suggested. With so many competing forces simultaneously pulling on caregivers, especially in the emergency department and intensive care units, standardized checklists can help us not overlook or forget critical steps in our patient care. They can be vital tools in support of critical thinking.

Process measures are the most common measurements providing data at a single hospital or even hospital system level. They have the advantage of being concurrent, easily measurable, and, after analyses (the fourth **W, WHY**), often will lead directly to improvement activities.

Organizations have increasingly committed to quality and safety goals that are almost always associated with staff incentive programs of some consequence. Tens of thousands of dollars can be a powerful tool in energizing commitment to safety and quality standards. These bonuses sometimes become the primary focus for staff and potentially undermine other motivations.

The ultimate driver should often be personal accountability and commitment to the patients we serve.

The Intuitive Opportunity Index helped us select and prioritize several quality indicators. Appropriate radiological procedure and length of stay are primarily process measurements. The sepsis data is compiled from both process and outcome measures. The bundle process measures are aimed mainly at the initial recognition and emergency treatment of the septic patient. Outcome measures in sepsis patients are reflected in the overall death rate and readmission rate.

Process measures may also be found on national data sets. Leapfrog (https://www.leapfroggroup.org), for example, has data primarily from four types of measurements in two categories. Leapfrog is a national organization that compiles data from about four thousand hospitals. It started as an organization that evaluated and published, in the lay literature, survey data about intensive care unit safety and capabilities.

✳ Leapfrog has morphed into a published compilation of multiple surveys and data-based patient and hospital statistics. Leapfrog is undoubtedly not the only non-governmental agency that endeavors to provide the public with information that allows for better decision-making about their care choices. It has, however, continued to improve its methodology since its inception. One clear example of this is that individual hospital survey questions that were initially voluntary are now subject to audit by the organization. In answering the question "What is the span of coverage in the ICU by intensivists?" each facility now must provide evidence in documented scheduling and timely response rates of the critical care intensivist physicians.

✳ Leapfrog provides a well-publicized, nationally accepted grade for hospitals. This is a precious tool in the armamentarium for *patient decisions* and *provider selection*. It includes information that allows the patient to take more control of their health care process. This is an essential key for patients in navigating the complex organizational structure of the current modern health care model.

Leapfrog and similar organizations have produced increasingly accurate and detailed information that promotes serious self-assessment of hospitals and their care. Utilizing the Leapfrog data, understanding how it compares to similar hospitals nationally, and then analyzing it becomes a serious tool for *process improvement* in a facility. There currently are multiple facilities that do not utilize Leapfrog and similar national data because they focus on *incentive-based* local process measures.

The first category in Leapfrog is *process and structure* measures. Much of this is survey-based and reflects the organization's safety culture. The second very prominent feature of Leapfrog is the inclusion of patient survey data: HCAHPS. Since 2008, this matrix has presented a twenty-nine-item, standardized publicly reported patient's perspective of hospital care and *directly reflected patient satisfaction.* This data comes from surveys given to patients and their families immediately following hospitalization. The surveys themselves are based on strenuous evaluation of hospital and staff attributes that patients can evaluate. For example, questions aim to express the satisfaction that patients feel about their communication with doctors and the nursing staff. The questionnaires are sent out quickly after discharge, and their return rate is reasonable, and they are statistically significant.

As always with survey data, there is much discussion about its validity, but it has become a stable part of the quality of the medical care evaluation process. This is important because the patient is the consumer and the end product. Patient satisfaction is no longer the purview of consumer-based rating enterprises such as Yelp but an increasing part of the backbone of evaluating the total value of medical services.

✦ In internal medical/hospital system surveys, when the patients are asked about the most crucial element in their care, the most overwhelming feature is *communication* and listening from the patient's point of view. Leapfrog does an excellent job at culling out patients' responses to specific questions about communication, such as the evaluation by the patient of their receipt and understanding of discharge instructions.

✖ There are articulated suspicions by hospitals and providers that these HCAHPS surveys do not really provide a significant reflection of overall medical services. However, they suggest that the increase in direct communication barriers attributed to technological advances in medicine negatively impacts the patient's sense of caring. It is hard to imagine that the insertion of the computer between the caregiver and the patient, the increasing introduction of noncontact interactions mediated through telehealth devices, the reliance on sophisticated testing rather than physical examination, and the multiplicity of caregivers involved in every case don't seriously impact communication. ✓✓ Patients are increasingly frustrated with the lack of one-on-one communication and the limited time that medical and support staff actually listen to their input and questions.

In addition to HCAHPS data reflective of how our patients feel about their care, it underscores that medical care must be a contract between the care team and the patient. It is essential that the patient not be a passive receiver of medical services. Much of the responsibility for the success of medical care depends on both the care receiver and the caregiver.

As the theme of personal accountability for the doctor and all the souls on the care team hopefully has been apparent throughout these pages, so should the corollary that the patient is responsible for their own care. This is obvious for things like following instructions, a rational diet and activities, and rigorous compliance with medication and rehabilitation requirements. In addition, the patient must adhere to follow-up reappointments and revisits. Compliance is far from 100 percent. The more significant the illness or injury, the more psychologically and physiologically committed the patient must be to their own care.

Utilizing information from HCAHPS not only assists patient choices in their selection of hospitals or doctors but allows them to have an increasing element of control over their care. This also symbolizes and publicizes integrating the patient's amygdala and feelings about their care.

Patients appreciate the publication of data that reflects their satisfaction and dissatisfaction with their care. It also encourages them to look more closely at the human elements of care and how to make their emotional and psychological elements of care a priority.

Having participated in several *patient safety committees* has enhanced my perspective. These groups are made up of former patients who ideally represent a cross-section of the geographic market. They report on their own care and input from other members of the community, not the technical aspects but elements such as communication and caring and even such things as cleanliness and noise levels.

- "The nurses are lovely. They do a great job. But they seemed overworked."

- "Every time I fall asleep, someone is bothering me and doing something in my room."

- "They ask my name and birthdate every time. You think they would know me by now."

- "At night, when I am sleeping, they place that linen cart in the hall by my room and has this loud squeaky wheel."

- "The other patient in my room moaned all night."

These comments and many more, sometimes amusing and sometimes very serious, bring home the hospital experience through the patient safety committee to the hospital executives and managers. The former patients and community members bring a vital and valuable perspective to the meetings. They are always taken seriously, and respectfully as the community members donate their time and deserve responses and solutions when available. This is another example of a functioning *team* that can accept new members and opinions.

The government has chosen a handful of diagnoses that represent the safety of care of our patients. Many of these PSI (patient safety indicators) make up the third element of Leapfrog. For the most part, these are chosen from a list of patients who die or have significant complications while in the acute care setting.

Safety and quality overlap consistently, but the former represents a low index of complicating or *Harm* events that are thought to be preventable. In contrast, quality focuses on large statistically valid data sets. Quality data stems from in-depth analysis of processes and outcomes that can lead to the overall improvement of patient care. The approach to both safety and quality has always been similar. They have given birth to burgeoning specialists such as IHI (see Craigs Clapper's *Zero Harm*), who have refined the approach to harm events, their understanding, and the path to preventing them in the future. Their and others' work has birthed HRO (high-reliability organizations), which has been successful in the broad-spectrum education of staff to prevent Harm events.

Through a meticulous severity grading process and subsequent event analysis (previously root cause analysis), the selection of these Harm events brings to the table individuals involved in an event and folks with the authority and resources to develop fixes. One of the main goals is to support the caregivers involved in an event and have them be fully engaged in the improvement work.

✴   HRO (High-Reliability Organization) study points out that most Harm events were not caused by a lack of knowledge but by a series of connected circumstances, such as deviating from established protocols. If one looks carefully at the pre-HRO installation, action plans suggested by most organizations in response to Harm events were commonly "educate the staff," or even worse, punish involved staff. A better understanding of which organizations are currently teaching has more to do with a "thoughtful pause" before actions, dependence on the engineered process, and the support of critical thinking.

✴   This is best characterized by the *time-out* done in the operating room before any procedure. This articulates to all team members required to participate core information such as correct patient, correct operative site, correct operation, and the presence of appropriate consents, the necessary materials and equipment. It also reinforces the theme articulated in our quality discussion of personal attention, commitment, and accountability (The buck stops here.).

✴   HRO looks at a single case in great depth and is not swayed by statistical considerations. "We never or rarely see this complication, or it is only one out of a thousand" holds no water when looking at serious complications. The airline industry, naval aviation, and nuclear power have seen remarkable improvements based on the HRO approach. Standardization, a powerful HRO theme, is an increasing" mantra" for medical organizations. However, some recent aviation losses underscore how uncertainty, such as we see in medicine, can complicate highly reliable organizations and how much ultimately comes down to personal accountability and commitment (Further discussion of this will come in the section: **Fifth W: WHAT are we doing about it.**.

Taylor McCaffery is a sixty-seven-year-old man with a history of multiple episodes of urinary tract infection. His primary care physician has sent him to see a urologist on several occasions, who recommended regimens of broad-spectrum antibiotics. The urologist also recommended prostate surgery for an enlarged gland, but Taylor refused since he did not want to contemplate the possible loss of his sexual capabilities. After retirement, his self-image suffered severely, and his continued "dating "was imperative to his psychological health.

Most recently, Taylor suffered several bouts of watery diarrhea, the second bout so severe that he was sent to the emergency department by his primary physician. When seen in the ED, he appeared toxic, febrile, and dehydrated. He had no further diarrhea but was admitted for IV hydration and antibiotics.

✶ ✼ Patients like Mr. McCaffery are at extremely high risk for a bacterial infection called C. diff. (Clostridioides difficile). This opportunistic organism thrives in the GI tract when the normal bacterial flora there is suppressed by antibiotics. Although most physicians are pretty sensitive to the risk of C. diff, this patient, like many others, was treated over an extended period with multiple courses and types of antibiotics, complicated by several doctors treating him simultaneously.

Cultures of his diarrhea revealed C. diff. This data was collected and collated by the government and then used by Leapfrog as part of its *outcome* measures in calculating the hospital's safety grade.

✔ This C. diff calculation is understandable as the overuse of antibiotics is something each hospital must be responsible for. In McCaffery's case, the treating hospital had only three cases of C. diff reported for a calendar year. Relative to a small regional hospital volume, the percentage of involved patients reported on national scorecards was more significant than the national average contributing to an overall decreased hospital grade. The further question that this case presents is related to the responsibility for his medication overuse. Was his C. diff caused by his repeated outpatient use of broad-spectrum antibiotics, was it because he did not wish to follow the recommendations of his physicians to have prostate surgery, or was it attributable to the hospital encounter and the IV antibiotics used to treat the serious infection?

These questions further illustrate why national grading systems are only excellent starting places for process improvements. The grade for C. diff at McCaffery's hospital was only the first step in a robust quality process.

Except for some notable exceptions, *process measures* are the primary data source at the hospital/system level. National organizations usually provide outcome measures with access to governmental data. For Leapfrog, the outcome data comes primarily from the CMS (Centers for Medicare & Medicaid Services) and is reproducible on multiple national agency reports. This data comes from *codes*, not from the actual review of patients or even a careful analysis of chart documentation. These codes are derived more and more from computer-assisted programs that rely on word recognition. As AI evolves in this field, coding accuracy continues to improve under the watchful eye of seasoned coders with a considerable amount of education and experience. Nevertheless, validation becomes critical and underscores **What the data is** must be seen as a first step, not an endpoint.

In the middle 2000s, the IHI (Institute for Healthcare Improvement), under the leadership of Dr. Don Berwick, started to mainline what at that time was known as the *triple aim*. This was an attempt at optimizing health care by prioritizing three aims specifically rather than embracing a more global, less focused approach. The three dimensions described were as follows:

- Improving the patient experience of care (including quality and satisfaction)

  o Motivating and engaging patients to play an active role in their care improves outcomes and safety.

- Improving the health of populations

o Preventing and managing prevalent, costly, and chronic diseases.

- Reducing the per capita cost of health care

  o Reducing resource utilization and readmissions while assuming more significant risk.

✦ It was reported that the US health system was the costliest globally, accounting for 17 percent of the gross national product with an estimate that it would be nearly 20 percent by 2020. Most health care systems providing inpatient and outpatient medical care were not accountable for the elements of the triple aim, and efficiency and finance were not accepted as essential elements of quality and safety.

With the passage of the *Affordable Care Act* emphasizing quality care at lower cost, the IHI expanded the Triple Aim to include provider satisfaction and rebranded it as the *Quadruple Aim.*

Improving provider Satisfaction

  o Providing access to tools and resources to address provider burden and burnout

This last additional focus is undoubtedly very timely, considering the stress and personal risk that Covid has added to the medical workplace. The Quadruple Aim (74) has become one of the significant drivers for collecting accurate outcome measures that drive the journey toward safety, efficiency, and quality care, reflected in the increasing availability of published national data.

One of the more creative governmental approaches for focusing on cost, quality, and safety is Value-Based Purchasing. VBP is a national program (CMS) highlighting how the government utilizes data to functionalize *pay for performance.* VBP is the only program with a potential incentive payment based on performance and a hefty penalty attribute. CMS's other two data-based programs are HRRP (*thirty-day readmissions to an acute care hospital*) *and HACRP (hospital-acquired conditions)* such as in-hospital C. difficile diarrhea. Lately, additional programs are being incorporated into penalties for hospitals, such as EDAC (extra days in acute care), which counts any bounce back to inpatient or outpatient hospital facilities, such as an ED visit within the thirty-day time frame.

⁎ VBP holds back 2 percent of *all Medicare payments* to all hospitals. This is then possible to earn back as enhanced payments to a hospital the following year. The process is *competitive* based on the achievement levels of a hospital in four categories.

- Clinical care

  o Thirty-day mortality of acute MI

  o Heart failure thirty-day mortality

  o Pneumonia thirty-day mortality

  o COPD thirty-day mortality

  o Arthroplasty hip/knee complication rate

- Person and community engagement

  o The Quality of the Communication between doctors and nurses with patients

  o The Responsiveness of the hospital staff to patient calls and needs

  o The Communication about medications and the cleanliness and quietness of the hospital

  o The effectiveness of Discharge information

  o The evaluation of Care transition and the overall rating of hospitals

- Safety Data

  o Catheter-associated UTI

  o Central line-associated bloodstream infection C.Diff

o   MRSA bacteremia

o   Surgical site infection (SSI) abdominal hysterectomy

o   SSI colon surgery

- Cost reduction

o   Medicare spending per beneficiary (projected under 0.9873/$1.000)

A facility scoring in the top tenth percentile can get an additional 3.5 percent over the "reimbursed" 2 percent. A hospital with Medicare payments of $ 75,000,000 would then get other Medicare payments of 5.5 percent: $4,125,000. The natural beauty of VBP from the government's point of view is the competitive aspects and the incentive payments that come from the pool of penalties from the non-rewarded hospitals. This type of data impacts health care decision-makers and facilitates focus and resources on Quadruple Aim. It also contributes to the conversation with clinical people about the need to incorporate efficiency into the quality.

The data for VBP and the other pay-for-performance programs comes from coding and billing information for three of the measures. The fourth measure, community engagement, is derived from survey information. The number of surveys returned by patients leaving hospitals and outpatient departments is surprisingly stout and strongly statistically significant. These surveys represent an opportunity to get feedback from patients regarding the human aspects of care they are met with daily. The surveys give us the best look at the interaction between the patient and the caregivers. It evaluates communication, caring, and continuity of care that may be lost in our modern health care system.

All the sections have point totals that are based on national averages. To underscore this point, the Leapfrog score and the CMS star rating score are all competitive and not based on fixed preconceived data goals.

VII.
THE FOURTH W, WHY
(ANALYSIS OF DATA)

The most concerning issue about the current overwhelming data streams, besides getting lost and not prioritizing resources, is that it is very seductive as an endpoint. Data is appealing, it is sexy, it has helped us speak a common language, it has helped us develop an image, and in some ways, it cuts through problems very simplistically. When I stood before large executive groups, I would say 17 percent is not the answer. As you can imagine, there was a mixed response. "It is if it's our goal," or "Is it better or worse than it was?" Even the most valid, current, and prioritized data is only a road sign. It doesn't even tell us if we are on the correct path.

On the other hand, data does tell us where there may be significant opportunities, either by comparison with other health organizations or hospitals or even about individual patients. Once we follow the quality cascade, collect and collate the data, then validate, prioritize, and study, we finally can settle into discovering **WHY** the data exists. The following are some fundamental steps in data analysis.

- Reach out to whatever agency, organization, or operation that is publishing data and

    o get the most current data. This may be non-finalized or rough data, but studying it may fast-track responses. Dealing with data that is either months old or, at worst, years old doesn't help evaluate the current process. Dedicating resources to analyze or fix apparent situations for which time and effort have already been alleviated makes little sense.

- o obtain, if possible, a list of the specific patients upon which the data is based. Whether we are dealing with one or two instances, it is exceedingly helpful in deploying resources despite the statistical percentage.

- o Initiate In-depth study of specific patients that allows for in-depth analysis from a safety and quality perspective.

- Dialogue directly with either the government (CMS) or reporting agencies. In many cases, this will reveal the basis of data collection and may prove helpful in more in-depth case analysis. There seems to be an increase in willingness within agencies to engage with local clinical specialists.

- Develop a close working relationship with the coders, either those working for contracted operations or homegrown. Most coders work from home, which restricts developing a more intimate team relationship. Working collaboratively is highly productive and has been demonstrated to improve coding accuracy, which helps both the financial and quality goals.

- Do not abandon, either in person or telephonically, the need to have a personal dialogue that focuses on education, awareness, and information sharing with the team responsible for this stream of information.

- Do not abandon the responsibility for coding to contracted agencies. Some of these groups are excellent but need a review of their in-depth case review. This can be done but usually requires personnel who have exceptional expertise in coding and the dedicated time to review the medical record comprehensively. This is impossible to do at a 100 percent level. A list of "high priority" cases should be referred to the internal expert coders for review before the patient cases are referred to the billing office.

- Available in almost real-time now is specific selected data that can give us trend results, hordes of valuable information about our processes, and detailed information that can even impact the patient still under our care. We need to know the **WHY** of the data based on careful analysis and comprehensive observations.

The fourth **W**, **WHY**, starts to give us actionable information. However, it is not only the in-depth facts of a case or cases that analysis provides, but it is also the opportunity to integrate further the caregiver, the bedside "doer," in the process of improvement.

It is critically important to investigate the perspective of the people involved in the care process, not in general terms, but grounded in the care of the specific cases where opportunities exist for improvement. This must be accomplished thoughtfully and carefully. Not only is it the sharing of information in a safe environment, but it must reinforce the accountability of the participants without undermining them.

A simplistic but telling example of the need for staff involvement is the data on *efficient radiology* from the CMS star report. This data is specifically about the potential redundancy and safety issues that arise from using two exams rather than a single exam. This is due to the use of contrast material separately from the exam without contrast, requiring two studies. This results in two exposures to radiation and double-billing from the government's point of view. When the data due to this redundancy first became available in one hospital, several postulated theories could explain the need for two exams.

The first theory was this particular radiology location was the primary referral for hematology/oncology patients, and the use of both procedures assisted staging of cancer. The radiologists also claimed they reviewed all the orders for efficacy. The hospital accepted these explanations rather than get embroiled in second-guessing physician ordering practices and those of the radiologist's judgment of necessity. This stimulated healthy discussion until the following audited results were reported, only to show that the rate of double exams continued to be five times higher than the national average.

At that point, the analysis kicked into another gear. And each patient was looked at in-depth, and the multiple processes were followed up in great detail. The radiologists were still convinced that their screening process was such, that only appropriate orders were going through uncontested, and that a duplicate or excessive patient order was not being charged.

A quality team prioritized this data utilizing the intuitive opportunity index since the points projected on national scorecards would have significantly impacted the overall CMS star grade because the deviation of the score from national average data was so dramatic. When the team investigated from step one, the initiation from the hematology/oncology office, where many of these with and without orders were supposedly initiated, they were surprised by what they found. For the most part, the physicians in the oncology practice only ordered a CT (Computed Tomography) and the site rather than a more specific request. The front office person was the individual formally requesting the study, and she said, "I have always ordered both with/without." When we asked the hem/oncology physicians to review the orders, the majority, we were told, did not need both studies.

When we took this ordering information to the radiologists, they were highly shocked. They admitted since the pattern with the heme/oncology group was always to have the radiologic study on cancer patients with/without, they did not question the appropriateness of the studies.

The above is a quick summary of the significant time dedication and personal discussion with the physicians involved, reviewing the national data and results. It illustrates how habit and assumption could be at the basis of some ongoing patient care issues. It also shows the need to involve the "players" when looking to understand the operations of care segments. Making assumptions by only looking at the data may lead to a serious miscalculation.

The **WHY**, in this case, was due to bad habits and the lack of accountability for the ultimate decision-making by many professional individuals in the process stream. Unfortunately, this is not uncommon. It occurs when motivated individuals defer to other people in the stream or who are once removed from the direct impact. As a chief nurse at one of my hospitals was fond of saying, "No one comes to work planning on doing a bad job or making mistakes." For the most part, radiologists represent a group of highly qualified well-trained and experienced care providers that no longer touch or very rarely interact directly with patients but defer this to other practitioners in the stream. Increasingly, technology or autonomous programs do the lion's share of contact.

Today at the facility under discussion, the number of CT scans with and without is approximately 50 percent below the national average, changing from around 26 percent of the studies to less than 5 to 6 percent. This positively impacts the ultimate national grade, financial aspects, and the potential waste of resources of double studies. Most importantly, as a safety measure, it has reduced the risk to patients by significantly decreasing their radiation exposure.

The "with and without" discussion in highly visible radiological procedures is simplistic modeling of **WHY** the data happens. The material is much more complex and involved in the following examples utilizing readmissions and severe sepsis

We have discussed the distinction between process and outcome data, but the former needs to be looked at carefully to understand outcomes from a **WHY** point of view.

✴ When asking questions about the initial treatment of sepsis in the ED, we want to determine when certain things are done or not done. Most facilities have very structured programs to ensure compliance with a standardized process. This has been automatized, utilizing computerized electronic health records to include alarms and drop-down menus that don't allow progressive steps in patient care until "due diligence" is accomplished. Being asked to specifically check for allergies before being able to order any medications is an example of this.

✴ This is the area where Dr. Gawande's checklist manifesto can be quite helpful. The standardized approach helps ensure that vital steps are not missed or forgotten. It should be understood that this mandatory checklist is increasingly necessary for the frequently chaotic situations that sick and dying patients present.

Clinical judgment may be the most common pressing issue that is looked at in retrospect, sometimes even in a court of law. However, it is the overlooked, forgotten processes, or deviations from the protocol that are the most common "mistakes." This digression from protocols is often the **WHY** that explains the problematic quality and safety data.

When clinical care is looked at from a safety perspective, the focus is usually on those patients where significant "harm" has occurred. When looked at from a quality perspective, it is to characterize how patients are cared for utilizing "best practice." What percentage of the time did we hit a clinical process goal, like what percentage of patients received a flu shot during their stay in the acute setting?

Rose Jones was a sixty-nine-year-old who had increasing knee pain and swelling exacerbated by her Pilates and yoga four times per week. Dr. Jules admitted her for knee replacement surgery. The care of patients with this type of surgery has changed significantly over the last five years. The technical aspects of this and other orthopedic procedures have been refined and are now typically an outpatient procedure or, at most, one-day hospitalization (characterized as an outpatient in a bed by Medicare).

Rose had an uncomplicated surgery, but she complained of significant pain as she awakened from anesthesia in the recovery room. She was given the pain medication, an opioid, as proscribed by her doctor. She fell back to sleep and was aroused only briefly when her surgeon came to see her, looked at her dressing, and approved her transfer to the medical-surgical unit. On arrival on the medical-surgical floor, she thrashed in pain, and the nurse repeated the dose of the same pain medication she had received in the recovery room. Rose quieted down immediately, and after making sure she was comfortable in bed, the nurse went to care for another patient. When the nurse returned to the room fifteen minutes later, Rose had evidence of vomitus around her mouth and was not breathing. A code blue was called, but despite vigorous resuscitation, Rose was pronounced dead.

Death is not uncommon in a hospital setting, but the unexpected death after a procedure, particularly an elective one, is intolerable. From a safety point of view, Rose's case went through rigorous review. There were multiple crossroads where strict guidelines were not adhered to. Numerous people did not follow specific "in-stone" procedures either centrally involved in her care or had peripheral opportunities to impact the outcome. The in-depth case review uncovered decisions made by members of the staff that increased the probability of an untoward outcome. No one, in this case, came to work with the thought of doing a poor job or putting a patient at risk. The involved caregivers took responsibility for the outcome during the meeting, but all initially viewed others' roles as significantly responsible.

The safety leadership's job was to focus the conversation away from blame, support the involved staff, and move toward understanding and action to prevent future similar circumstances. The immediate necessity was to inform the family of the outcome and the possible reasons for the unfortunate results. Candor is one of several processes that directs and assists staff in patient notification, explanation, and support after a Harm event. However, awkward, there was a high probability that all parties and organizations involved would share the blame.

From a *quality* point of view, the preceding root cause analysis initially took center stage, but then the focus became increasingly data-centric. How often do steps in the safe patient care process, post knee surgery, get missed, and **WHY**? This required not only an in-depth study of Rose's case but of all similar surgeries, especially those *without* complications. They are looking for opportunities to improve care, not just looking at ways to avoid disasters. Regional and national data is beneficial in these circumstances as it disallows hiding behind local non-statistical idiosyncrasies. This is assisted by knowing about other institutions, processes, and outcomes. The staff is trained to ask **WHY** as they "peel the onion" of complex behaviors and understand the essential elements of intricate care patterns.

After an in-depth in-person case review, the medical record is an excellent place to start looking for the **WHY**. As mentioned, now coding is utilized nationally and locally as a system to look at large data sets. Once alerted by the codes, many hospital facilities now use senior internal coders to review the initial codes. There are only a small number of patient cases that highlight documented issues. This allows for a more comprehensive chart audit and some opportunity to reach out to clinicians for better or additional documentation. This secondary review follows strict compliance standards and must be done before a patient is discharged from a facility. Patient charts that don't meet standards or clinical goals have a robust clinical review. Part of this is to look for **WHY** and opportunities for improvement. It also provides senior clinical leaders with an in-depth, focused examination of selected issues. In the detailed study of these cases, leadership engagement is imperative when entering the fifth **W** (**What** will we do about it?).

Selected clinical records are then brought to clinical committees for discussion. The entire team has the advantage of a timely review of specific patient care, and all are invited to add their perspectives. However, this is often time-consuming and sometimes disruptive to the intense daily activities in an acute care setting. Yet, it prioritizes the intense interrelated activities of the team and further personalizes and reinforces accountability.

- Specifically, in the care of the sepsis patient, there are multiple focus areas.

    - Early recognition. Both at triage in the ED and the hospitalized patient, a compilation of patient data and *intuitive analytics* rings bells to *alert the possibility* of sepsis. Time may be the most significant factor in the successful treatment of a patient with sepsis.

    - Once recognized or suspected, vigorous early treatment with *fluids and antibiotics* is critical. Current literature has challenged and mitigated the amount of fluids and their duration. Still, there is little doubt that both of these elements are necessary considerations as early as possible in the patient's course.

    - Careful *patient monitoring* should go without saying, but as every patient is defined by unique clinical circumstances and physiology, frequent reevaluation is required.

- The *diagnostic evaluation* must move rapidly and includes blood tests and cultures.

- Sepsis, even when treated effectively early, often requires significant hospitalization and prolonged recovery. Patient *education* and post "discharge" planning must be accomplished repeatedly and early on in the process of inpatient care. *Prioritization* of the neediest patients significantly assists in resource management.

- Some patients will develop severe *sepsis while hospitalized* for other illnesses, and early recognition and systemized approaches for the care of these inpatients must exist.

- *Care across the continuum* is established with discharge phone calls, Home Health visits, "Meds to Beds" (ensuring appropriate follow-up outpatient medications go home with patients), post-acute facility placement, and outpatient physical therapy.

- Medical *follow-up visits* need to be established before discharge, ideally within three to five days. Patients should leave the hospital with an appointment that they have agreed to. The medical record should be available through the electronic health record in the hands of the local provider at the time of a patient's re-visit.

- Sepsis patients have a very high rate of seven- to thirty-day *readmissions*. Many may seek further care within seventy-two hours. A well-established system must exist to care for these patients efficiently.

If there are multiple comprehensive processes to foster quality and safety practices, **WHY** do errors, omissions, and non-adherence to accepted protocols occur? Some of these events occur because of an almost infinite variety of circumstances. Few patients with acute appendicitis, for example, are the same. The symptoms and time of onset vary. The character of the pain is highly subjective. The age and sex of the patient may alter a classic presentation. The possibility of concurrent pregnancy or other GYN-related illnesses complicates both diagnosis and treatment approaches. The presence or lack of comorbidities; medication, drug, alcohol, and cigarette smoking history; a history of prior abdominal surgery; complicating social issues, including the patient's language skills, add complexity and uncertainty.

We often would like to explain some adverse outcomes or circumstances because of the expanding workloads of the staff, as well as the loss of focus that something like Covid in our midst causes. Because of the risk of infection during the pandemic, the personal risk alone that each staff member has faced can cause a loss of focused attention. The wild changes in the hospital's physical plant and standard patterns of care and the almost weekly changes in protocols caused by the pandemic have had the potential to increase errors and omissions. During the same period as the Covid pandemic surges, and for other reasons as well, hospitals have faced overwhelming patient numbers and even obvious overloads. These circumstances are potentially on the table as reasons for **WHY** things happen.

There have been significant studies on the causality of **WHY** "bad" things happen in the patient safety realm. Kathleen Sutcliff, in her book, *Still Not Safe* (75), and Craig Clapper in *Zero Harm*, take the pioneering work of James Reason and utilize it to establish a classification grid for understanding the **WHY** of medical errors. "Human beings experience three types of errors: skill-based, rule-based and knowledge-based" (76).

- Skill-based: A well-established pattern in the brain from practice and repetition. Distraction, fatigue, and loss of attention are significant contributors, but for the most part, errors occur in less than 1/1000 tasks. In the following table, these are in the consciousness error category.

- Rule-based: Education or experience provide the operating principle or rule, and these are subject to more common errors, particularly in medicine, about 1/100.

- Knowledge-based: New or unfamiliar situations cause about 30-plus percent of errors. These fall into the competency error category in the following table.

In the following table, errors in communication, critical thinking, and compliance are sometimes rule-based and knowledge-based (77).

Individual Failure Modes [(78) p. 103]

Category	Percent
Competency (knowledge & skill)	15.1
Consciousness. (attention on task)	11.4
Communication (information processing)	9.6
Critical Thinking (cognitive processing & decision making)	39.7
Compliance (including normalized deviance)	24.1

In thinking about this information, it is reasonable to question, what is the denominator in these statistics. Does the denominator count every medication usage, every meal and drink, diagnostic test, every change of rooms, every time the patient uses the bathroom or walks the halls, and every directed communication . . .? You get my drift.

This discussion is not aimed at invalidating or changing the focus from the hundreds of thousands of reported medical errors in hospitals each year, but rather the importance of the significance of the *study of each case* and the investigation of **WHY**. The starting point is the larger **WHY** that an FMEA (Failure Mode & Effects Analysis) provides.

FMEA was initiated in the military in the 1940s and is an organized step-by-step approach to identifying design failures. It is highly structured and managed, producing a grading system that helps prioritize solutions. It is one of several current programs utilized by hospital safety experts to understand better and implement change. The FMEA process helps not only understand problematic issues but organize action. There is a significant history in most organizations of thinking and discussing problems and not enough focus on the path necessary for doing something. FMEA has this feature at its core.

The Rose Jones case of unexpected death following orthopedic surgery, described previously, puts it into the failure modes category of critical thinking and processing. The nurses involved were well trained and experienced. They knew existing protocols and policies relative to opioid usage and dosing. The vigorous analysis that followed was framed in a process called just culture (This will be discussed in more detail in the fifth W **WHAT**.). It was clear that the nursing staff was trying to meet the patient's needs, who was crying uncontrollably in pain.

x   The involved nursing staff's significant biases contributed to their decision-making. In their nursing training, Pain was made the *fifth vital sign*, which put untoward focus on controlling the pain. Although subsequently deleted, the emphasis on pain control and the human nature to stop suffering is a powerful motivator to push the limits of medications to treat acute pain. Not only was Rose's death unacceptable, but it had the potential to destroy several nursing careers.

> "Working in a Just Culture means more security around your decisions. It means recognizing that humans aren't perfect and that when you make a mistake, you are going to be embraced in the process of trying to understand why the error was made rather than be punished for your mistake". (Paul LeSage, SG Collaborative Solutions, LLC, working at Brigham and Women's Faulkner Hospital)

Critical thinking is responsible for the largest category of "mistakes "and perhaps answers **WHY** these errors are so pervasive in the medical field. We are humans taking care of humans in an arena of complexity, uncertainty, and variability. Whether supported by paper or computer checklists, processes and protocols are considerably helpful in standardizing and enforcing behaviors. However, the bottom line; is compassionate care happens at the physical interface between caregiver and patient.

Critical thinking takes time and is arguably the most crucial element in decision-making. As discussed in earlier chapters, this decision-making is ideally balanced between algorithm, emotional intelligence, and intuition. Our daily lives, particularly in medicine, are a composite of small and large decisions that directly impact our patients and colleagues. These decisions may be straightforward, such as following protocols or checklists. They may depend on evaluating data and situations, collating information from multiple sources or individuals, and integrating one's intuition and gut-level responses.

Complex medical decisions are often made with *heuristic* behavior and bias at play, particularly under the stress of time and the critical nature of the judgment results. Daniel Kahneman says in <u>Thinking Fast and Slow</u>, "The technical definition of a heuristic [approach] is a simple procedure that helps find adequate, though often imperfect, answers to difficult questions" [(79) p. 98].

It is relatively straightforward to understand that a deviation from best practice or failure to comply with SOP (standard operating procedures) are errors, irrespective of whether they produce harm. The **WHY** here is asking for the reason for the missing considerations or steps that have been developed to reduce problematic results specifically. If a checklist is not followed or armbands are not thoroughly reviewed before medication administration, we may have only the first layer of **WHY**.

Remembering we are talking about humans taking care of humans, the human nature of the heuristic approach is somewhat responsible for our ability to prioritize decisions and rapidly implement the consequent action. Choosing those few elements that seem to be the most critical, particularly in an urgent or emergent situation, has long allowed first responders and others providing emergency care the ability to do the most important things first. This is the same rationale favoring *intuition* or pattern recognition in critical rapid decision-making. Before making a vital life-saving decision, it allows users not to wait for supporting evidence, lab tests, X-rays, or a comprehensive medical history.

Having practiced much of my life as an ER physician, with reliance on intuition and heuristic behavior with great success, it is difficult to come to grips with some inherent issues with this approach. Heuristic thinking leaves some potentially critical information on the table. Even more significant is the recurring theme of *bias*. It is impossible to leave bias out of the critical decision-making process. This includes the bias from our experiential history.

Unfortunately, the articulated thought "I have done it this way successfully so many times before" can compromise a complex and uncertain situation. A more subtle bias may exist: This may develop from deep-seated feelings about a patient, derived from social, religious, personality, smell, language, sexual orientation, or other clues.

In understanding the value of intuition and the potential negative aspects of bias, the sentinel work of James Reason in his book *Human Error* (80) introduced the deeply rooted psychological causes of human error. Addressing more than just failure modes and their analysis, Reason looks at all those features that can potentially cause Human Error, critical in a human-to-human business.

"Two conditions appear to be necessary for the occurrence of slips in action: the performance of some largely automatic task in familiar surroundings and a marked degree of attentional 'capture' by something other than the job at hand." (81) These are the circumstances the staff often finds themselves in a hectic acute care hospital setting.

Reason says, "The more routine the activity, the fewer the number of low-level control statements required to specify it. However, in novel activities, we are aware of the need to 'talk ourselves through" the actions. Under these circumstances, our activities are guided by the effortless yet computationally-powerful investment of conscious activities." (82) Craig Clapper in *Zero Harm* would characterize this as the need for a real or symbolic "time-out (83)."

A time-out has been the standard safety technique in the operating room and prior to procedures for many years in the hospital setting. The time-out enlists all parties involved, including doctors, nurses, and technologists, to ensure that the correct procedure is done on the right patient, proper location, that all components and materials are present, and that *consent* documentation is consistent with the situation. Every member of the team is accountable for all the elements. The compliance with time-outs outside of the operating room for minor procedures is less consistent and, unfortunately, is responsible for the occurrence of errors.

Guy Petersen was a seventy-nine-year-old man presenting to the emergency department with increasing shortness of breath and chest pain. Guy had worked as a contractor and had been extremely busy in the rapidly expanding home construction market. He recently left the job site earlier because of some tiredness and cough. He attributed his cough to his allergies which always got worse when his building sites produced a lot of dust. On the day of his ED visit, he had an increasing cough, shortness of breath, and significant chest discomfort.

On arrival, Guy struggled with breathing and was immediately triaged into a critical care bed. He had a red spotty rash, and decreased and noisy lung sounds both on the left and right on examination.

The patient was placed on oxygen and had an immediate EKG and a chest X-ray, and despite some mild protestations, he had an IV started and blood work sent for diagnostics. Although the oxygen helped, he continued to demonstrate shortness of breath and complain of pain. The X-ray revealed spotty lesions in both lungs and a significant pneumothorax on the right. The ED doctor had already set up the placement of a chest tube, as his exam revealed a hollowness and decrease of breath sounds in both lung fields. The X-ray confirmed a large air leak and a collapsed lung requiring urgent therapy. A chest tube was placed on the left, with surprisingly little response, and after rechecking the X-ray, the ED doctor noted the patient's primary pathology was on the right side. The chest tube was removed from the left and reinserted on the right, with an immediate change in the patient's condition. Significant air was removed from the patient's chest, and the right lung was able to reinflate.

"I feel much better, doc. Thanks," the patient exclaimed.

"We treated the air pocket that a leak in your lung created; now we need to admit you and figure out what the lesions in your lung are from so we can treat you," said the ED doctor.

"Do I have cancer, doctor?"

"That is a possibility, but I think you more likely have valley fever, so we need to rule that out. One step at a time."

"Thanks, doc. What is this, valley fever?"

"Valley fever comes from a fungus called coccidioidomycosis, which can be treated." The doctor paused for a minute and then said, "I do have to tell you that I put the tube on the left side of your chest at first, which I corrected immediately. We can talk more about that after getting you comfortable and in the intensive care unit."

"How could that have happened?" the patient asked with some confusion.

"You were struggling to breathe, and I wanted to get the chest tube in as quickly as possible to make you feel better. I was worried about the strain on your heart. I can only tell you this will become part of your record, and while you are here, other folks will talk to you and your family more about this and more about your diagnosis and therapy."

It should be noted that the doctor never verbalized that he made a mistake or was sorry about having to put two chest tubes in the patient. There is a thin line between the immediate notification to patients of errors and utilizing the language that reinforces litigation and liability.

This difficult conversation about a wrong side procedure would be supported through Candor, which would sponsor additional discussion, support for the patient and the family, and support for the staff involved in the actual incident. In the past, Guy Petersen's care would have been written off as "no harm, no foul" since the placement of a chest tube on the wrong side had no, or insignificant, complications.

Despite the lack of complications, the opportunity to discuss **WHY** such an event happened to Mr. Petersen provides a gift for the future. It is often the lack of conscious decision-making, a critical thinking pause, or the presence of situational bias that precedes human error in both standard and unique situations. The suspicion of Valley Fever, the uniqueness of its emergency rather than indolent presentation, and the patient's discomfort may have altered the medical team's focus from a well-recognized standard operating procedure.

Although less common than these errors in the absence of critical thinking, Reason defines knowledge-based issues as a common thread. His work, published in 1990, predated the medical computer era, the electronic health record, and immediate staff access to extensive supporting information. These developments have significantly decreased but not eliminated this error category. It is certainly possible to have the knowledge but not apply it situationally. This is more common when the appropriate questions are not asked, rather than not having the knowledge available.

As expressed by T. S. Eliot in the previously quoted poem, circumstances where there is lots of information, some conflicting, should progress to knowledge but stop short of wisdom, which comes from utilizing information, knowledge, and critical thinking.

James Reason goes on to list several knowledge-based pathologies: (84)

Selecting the wrong features of the problem space

- Being insensitive to the absence of relevant elements

- Confirmational bias

- Overconfidence and biased reviewing of plan construction

- Illusory correlation

- Halo effects

- Problems with causality and complexity with diagnosis in everyday life

The complexity of the psychology of human error as causal in medical mishaps helps us understand the **WHY** of the prominence of safety events. The omnipresence of bias, the utilization of repetition, and the complexity of human error causes contribute in part to what Wears and Sutcliffe describe as the basis for a" *plateau of improvement* in patient safety". (85) The tools for safety are in place. It is the absolute consistency of their use that is at stake.

> "I always check and mark for laterality before I do a proce-dure," the doctor who put the chest tube on the wrong side exclaimed, during the event analysis. "I have done chest tubes hundreds of times."

The emergency physician, and the team around him, treating Guy Petersen felt significant remorse about the wrong side chest tube. None of them came to work planning to make mistakes or do a lousy job. They relied too heavily on the procedural frequency and undervalued the necessity for critical thinking every time.

A great deal of effort has been put forward to place the critical deci-sion-maker into situations that, at least in part, can control the multiplicity of variables in health care. Standardization, checklists, protocols, built-in alarms in EHR, double checks, time-outs, and built-in redundancy are now all part of acute care in the hospital setting. Yet errors still are responsible for hundreds of thousands of poor outcomes and deaths, liability, and financial loss for organizations and individuals.

The direct loss of human life and limb has made decision-making at every level a key element in medicine. Other fields such as aviation and the nuclear power industry also have very visual and impactful evidence of this. The lessons learned, however, are also transferrable to many other fields. The dependency on technology and standardization cannot totally replace the decision-maker. This is particularly true as the decision becomes increasingly complex in situations of uncertainty and variability.

In the introduction to his book *How We Decide*, Jonah Lehrer (86) describes a harrowing event:

> I was flying a Boeing 737 into Tokyo International Airport when the left engine caught fire. We were at seven thousand feet, with the runway dead ahead and the skyscrapers were shimmering in the distance. Within seconds, bells and horns

blared inside the cockpit, warning me of multiple system failures. Red lights flashed all over the place. I tried to suppress my panic by focusing on the automated engine-fire checklist, which told me to cut off fuel and power to the affected areas. Then the plane began a steep bank. The evening sky turned sideways. I struggled to steer the aircraft straight . . .

I didn't know what to do . . . It was a hellish moment of indecision. Nervous sweat stung my eyes. My hands quivered with fear. I tried to think, but there wasn't time.

Lehrer ultimately tells us that the experience he related was in a simulator, although it seemed incredibly real. He uses this example of the need for balance between reason and listening to our emotions.

Decision-making in medicine, or other fields where critical outcomes are at stake, can be a blend of brain functions. The decision vortex mentioned earlier illustrates the functional makeup of critical thinking and decision-making. The OFC (orbitofrontal cortex) is responsible for integrating the emotions from the midbrain and amygdala [(87) Lehrer p. 18] which functionalizes the three elements of the decision vortex triangle.

My focus in decision-making has been in medicine, where morbidity and mortality closely follow when critical thinking fails to incorporate all brain elements. Recognizing these decision-making features is essential in the decisions themselves as well as for the executives, directors and managers responsible for daily critical decisions. Comprehending the importance of every decision and taking it personally is necessary for galvanizing staff to obtain the relevant data, all the inputs, and the consequences of the decision. No matter how truncated, utilizing a time-out allows for integrating multiple decision-making elements.

Understanding the data necessary to make judgments in life and death decisions is commonplace in medicine. It is critical in aerospace and nuclear power, but it is key to conclusions in many other fields.

In a recent article in Bloomberg Businessweek, "The pandemic has shut the door on the value of meticulous planning" (88). The corollary is the recognition of the fluidity of situations and the added complexity and uncertainty of moment-moment decision-making. Life and death might not be the only consequences of critical thinking failures, but millions of dollars and the health and welfare of communities may also hang in the balance.

Kahneman and Tversky focus on decision-making in economics, explicitly investing, and point out that human emotions and bias play a significant role even in projections, statistical probabilities, historical information, and trends.

✶ HROs (Highly Reliable Organizations) spend hundreds of thousands of dollars and vast amounts of staff time arguing that critical thinking is still the essential element of highly safe care in medicine and success in multiple other business ventures. How to instill the personal attachment and ownership at a midbrain level that leads to accountability and personal commitment in decision making is the question for the fifth **W** (**WHAT** we can do about it).

SAFETY AND QUALITY

When approached and asked, "What is the primary goal of your facility?" every hospital executive will answer, "Safety and quality for our patients." Although these are circles with significant overlap, the quest for these meritorious states of being and the seeking of the **WHY** is significantly different.

Finding those cases that have errors or even deviate significantly from best practice is done manually through relentless chart review, complaint investigation, information system technologies for voluntary reporting, and recently through technologies like *root trigger monitoring*.

Hospital rounds. Once the purview of only teaching hospitals, rounds daily incorporating the entire care team are commonplace. In addition to marking a patient's progress and discussing diagnosis and therapies, problems in care often come forward. These cases are then referred to a quality coordinator to review. These manual reviews are time-consuming but often reveal operational and critical decision-making information. Cases then can be referred to medical staff or hospital-based committees. This pathway is also open to referrals from multiple credible sources within the hospital community.

- **Complaint investigation**. Patient and family letters expressing concern or dissatisfaction about the care they received used to go to the dead letter office. Today they find their way immediately to the C-suite, where they are referred for investigation and, by rule, must be answered within a week. This process has enhanced the awareness of a continuous low level of areas of concern and relatively rapid response and resolution.

- **IVOS** (Incident Reporting System). This, and systems similar to it, are a repository of concerns entered into the electronic health care information system by anyone in the internal hospital community. They represent an extensive range of issues: staffing concerns, supply issues, behavior deviations, policy and procedure problems, and direct patient care issues. The strength of IVOS is that *anyone* can enter a topic. The weakness is it is voluntary for the most part. Data suggests that IVOS only lists about 20 percent of patient care concerns.

- **Augmented intelligence systems** (we don't like the term artificial intelligence). An excellent example of these systems is RTM (*root trigger monitoring*). These systems monitor the live electronic health record and, on the basis of selected triggers, will report within fifteen minutes deviations that might represent opportunities for improvement. An excellent example is reversal agents after patients leave the recovery room because of consciousness or breathing problems. These agents, such as naloxone, are used when the effects of opioid medications are excessive.

- The use of Naloxone in the post-operative areas is a trigger that can lead to immediate positive reactions in direct patient care. Its use also leads to the in-depth study of **WHY** an issue occurred and the subsequent opportunities for improvement. This data can be accumulated, collated, reported, and compared to other facilities. The strength of RTM is its immediacy and impact on ongoing patient care. The weakness of RTM is the need for enhanced resources for real-time surveillance and the follow-up of identified problems in care.

The safety discussion is monumental, based on the hundreds of thousands of medical errors reported yearly in the United States. The impact on patient lives, the personal liability of health care organizations and their personnel, and what it might mean professionally and financially are exceptionally weighty. The small number of these "errors," no matter how devastating, does allow for in-depth investigation.

Even actively utilizing *just culture*, the impact on the staff involved may be excruciating. Event analysis is "up close and personal" and demands intellectual and emotional accountability. Such errors have ended careers, made a long-term psychological impact, and are an indelible learning opportunity. The effect is long-lasting and unforgettable.

Another answer to the **WHY** of the Rose Jones case (the unfortunate patient who died after elective knee replacement) is no less forthcoming from the specifics of the case analysis and is still extremely difficult to pinpoint. One must truthfully question the culture of the hospital organization and the culture of the individual physicians and nurses involved. Has the pressure from governmental agencies to increase the efficiency of care for this select group of patients decreased safety precautions? Covid and its impact on basic nursing must be questioned. Did the bias for treating postoperative pain in a short-term admission impact critical decision-making? Were the nurses "burned out" by the unrelenting patients and problems that Covid presented to the hospital?

Based on the statistics, since Covid, on the number of qualified nurses leaving their jobs, burnout would be a significant possibility. The demands, the stress, and the fear that permeated the staff during the pandemic will continue to have a lasting impact. The fact that nurses, for a variety of reasons, can now demand higher salaries for their services is widely published. Still, it can only partly defer the current hospital environment's stress, risk, and increasing demands. Management is under fire to continue to provide a level of service without a significant increase in resources, which somewhat also alters the culture of human contact and caring. Ultimately this value starts to be eroded and cannot be repaired by dollars alone.

Physicians as well have found themselves working in an increasingly hostile environment. Trying to maintain their practice patterns and financial status during a pandemic, for many, has changed their patient commitment. When the nurses were asked about their lack of communication with the physician of record in the Rose Jones case, they replied, "He hates to be bothered." This, as can be imagined, discourages communication, which is the lynchpin of good safe care. This type of culture is much more difficult to "fix" than relying on processes and checklists in the long run.

The safety movement tends "to focus on the unusual, dramatic accidents or rescues" [(89) p. 43]. There is a significant crossover into risk management. Acknowledging events, communicating with patients and families, ultimately working with legal teams, and adjudicating liabilities have become a cottage industry.

There is a tremendous reliance on the work done in the airline industry, military aviation, and nuclear power in adopting methodology and understanding medical mishaps or near misses. None of these other industries have the statistical potential of mishaps, although one error can cause devastating calamity and death. The daily number of decisions and actions multiplied by the number of patients in the acute care setting statistically enhances error probability.

Although *safety and quality programs* are often lumped together and share the national stage, they overlap (as mentioned previously), but they have significant distinguishing differences. "In contrast to patient safety, the quality movement did not explicitly focus on harm or even errors. Rather it aimed at standardization, identification, and implementation of best practices, and <u>improving access to care and decreasing costs.</u> Substandard or less effective care was discouraged more because it was economically or clinically inefficient than because patients might be harmed" [(90) p. 42].

✳ Secondary to the understanding of the potential financial impact of quality, both the government and hospital systems recognized the need to resource quality programs. "They focused on the routine aspects of care, making sure ordinary care was delivered within well-defined standards. In contrast, safety advocates . . . tended to focus on the unusual, dramatic accidents or rescues" [(91) p. 43].

✳ Two areas that have seen a tremendous amount of focus in quality management are the care of the *sepsis patient and readmissions*. These fall into Wear and Sutcliff's description of "standard care," which has significant financial aspects and far-reaching patient care issues.

✳ In addition, both sepsis and readmission cases have multiple other reasons for aggressive clinical management.

- National volumes of hospital-specific data are immediately available.

- Copious state and national data are available.

- National standards for best practices are available.

- Both sepsis and readmissions have well-recognized process measures.

- Both sepsis and readmissions have well-recognized outcome measures.

- Data from both drive *penalty and incentive* programs.

- Data is apparent on many systems-wide hospital quality incentive programs.

- Data is used in multiple national data-based matrices.

- Data is used on multiple publicly reported. National grading sites.

- Sepsis and readmissions have a significant direct and indirect financial impact.

Initially, when quality management dug into sepsis and readmission data, there were multiple barriers to the effective use of this valuable information. Local hospital data was not treated statistically, was slow to be published, and was heavily based on tedious chart review. National data were often two to three years old and based entirely on coding. Leaders and decision-makers were only shown the **WHAT** data rather than the analyzed **WHY** data. It is only in the last few years, that timely and validated statistically significant data has been used to impact the immediate care of patients.

Balancing out the **WHAT** of all the system, governmental, and agency data that ultimately stems from patient chart documentation and coding and billing review, HCAPHS (hospital consumer assessment of healthcare providers and systems) allows us a selected but potentially in-depth review of the patient's perspective of their care. As discussed in the section on VBP (*value-based purchasing*), the survey measures reveal a great deal about the care we provide. Survey designs, although not perfect, try to avoid popularity and bias and shed light on the human elements of care. They are explicitly directed at representative aspects of communication. Patients repeatedly choose this communication as the number one element they believe is most important in their care. The patient wants to feel cared for, and as discussed, this element is essential in their care plan. If positive on a midbrain level, how the patient feels emotionally about their care team strongly reinforces their compliance to medication, behavioral adjustments, and overall getting well.

Although met with some hesitancy from staff about their meaningfulness, the surveys are our most consistent bridge to understand the human aspects of our care. As they represent 25 percent of our VBP (value-based purchasing) grade, organizations are forced to look at them seriously. This is fortunate as the organizational bias about data strongly favors numbers, grades, and percentiles to the more complex "softer" elements of patient perception. Psychologically, survey data has never had the same impact as numerical

✾ data. *Outcome data* is the "gold standard" because it is the ultimate measure of the efficacy of all our processes, operations, and resource deployment. Yet this data gives us very little insight into the **WHY** of human error or the commitment and accountability that support communication and trust at a very midbrain level.

Utilizing the surveys as a jumping-off point, several things assist in asking **WHY** a patient or patients feels a certain way about their care. One of the most compelling insights comes from reviewing the surveys for specific comments. Although this is difficult to standardize, it reveals much about our people and processes responsible for overall patient care. This also makes an excellent starting point for employing techniques of "**WHAT** can we do about it" that will be discussed more fully in the next section.

The review of the care of *sepsis patients* has provided a steady stream of data that has and continues to impact care positively. Most data streams have become increasingly current or even concurrent and continue to improve outcomes and impact the care of individual patients currently being treated.

Recalling the discussion about the patient Thomas Conner with sepsis, his case highlights an aggressive approach to his care and the concurrent collection of meaningful data. Thomas was our paddle ball player who got sepsis from a blister on his big toe. It should be mentioned, even if in passing, that Thomas also is representative of a group of patients who, despite their protestations, were saved by their spouse's determination.

Information about the best practice processes of care in sepsis patients and its outcome data have been analyzed from a **WHY** perspective. There is a patient-by-patient relentless pursuit of current opportunities that can improve the immediate care of active patients and supply clinically significant information about process improvement. In Thomas' case, his care met the timing of all the "bundle elements." We know that the sepsis data is very dependent on early recognition and aggressively timed treatment, and each process element is concurrently studied under the microscope. This is part of the process of data being carefully studied in many hospital systems.

Studies also show that the patient's understanding of their disease and comprehensive follow-up after hospital discharge are equally essential elements of care. This intensive search for **WHY** allows for continuous improvement activities at the level at which care is provided.

One of the critical lessons from this evaluation is that *continuity of care* is problematic in our current health care system. At least in part, readmission of our sepsis patients is responsible for approximately 30 percent of all our readmissions. Continuity was generally discussed previously in the "C" section but has specific relevance to sepsis. As laboratories that assist in the careful study of health care, sepsis and readmissions exemplify current care trends and reveal, unsurprisingly, the need to focus on the fifth **W, WHAT** we can do about it.

We have been through the first **W: WHAT** is our organization in terms of goals, culture, leadership, and mores? The second **W, WHY**, is a close look at why we are here as individuals, what we feel about ourselves and the organization we are part of. It also comprises understanding our emotions, biases, how we make decisions, and the impact on our midbrain which is all part of our performance and retention. The third **W** is about what we know about our operations. In medicine, this has been heavily focused on the oceans of data from a wide variety of sources that are now available for review. The fourth **W** is an understanding of **WHY** the data exists. The organizational and operational observations that stem from it become the first steps to process improvement.

WHAT CAN WE DO ABOUT IT?

The last **W**, which we are about to immerse ourselves in, is very personal and job-specific. As an emergency physician and hospital executive, my

WHAT list comes from my experiences and commitment to our patients. Yet I hope that the final **W**, as with the previous four **Ws**, can lead to perceptions applicable to a broader variety of industries where the human is still the key ingredient for success. VII. WHAT (what are the barriers, and what can we do about them?"

One of the most significant barriers to improving quality and safety is actually getting something done. Addressing the multiple opportunities that careful analysis and asking **WHY** errors happen and quality improvement doesn't isn't easy! Earlier I spoke a lot about the organizational culture of health care organizations and their stated goals. Safety and quality improvement are typically the mantra articulated through written and spoken company statements.

AUGMENTED INTELLIGENCE (AI)

One of the major approaches to the future of health care has been turning toward AI and the hope that health information systems and related technological advances would automatically improve both safety and quality. (92) The expectation that a standardized, simplified electronic system would eliminate or certainly reduce errors and improve performance has only been partially validated. It has replaced long-established cultural imperatives in many situations that traditionally incorporate human commitment, responsibility, accountability, and attachment to our patients.

I am not a naysayer about the actual and potential benefits of a well-designed and implemented health information system, but I am also quite concerned with the change of the focus of care to the machine rather than the patient.

When walking through the acute care wards, I see a considerable amount of clinicians' time and energy directed at the "box." The time actually interacting with patients directly can be measured in a few minutes. The physical exam is minimal and *biased* by information from diagnostic procedures and lab tests. Communication with the patient and the time for questions and answers are increasingly directed through the nursing staff.

The nursing and support staff spend much of their time clustered at workstations. To avoid congestion, WOWS (work stations on wheels) and follow the nurse in the hallway, at the nursing station or in the patient's room.

Documentation by the clinician has become the primary reflection of the quality of work done and compliance with accepted standards of care. It is also the basis for analytics and even more so for coding, which, as mentioned, is the basis for national comparisons and grades. Electronic chart documentation is also the basis for coding and the subsequent billing that relies directly on it. Much of the process depends directly only on what the physician documents into the record. Nursing, therapist, and technologist documentation is adjunctive but is used mainly to complement the doctor's charting and diagnosis. A reviewing third party, even a clinical one, cannot add, clarify, or interpret anything besides the physician's document.

This focus on "charting" and documentation has created a new industry of folks who constantly review active patient records that "query" physicians about documentation suggested by other elements in the chart, such as vital signs and lab and diagnostic tests. This is not only resource-heavy and time-demanding but psychologically pushes the clinical focus away from the patient. It is not difficult to see how taking care of the chart can sometimes rise in priority to taking care of the patient.

Another layer of chart review has now been developed because of the importance of the clinical record and its reflection on quality and safety. Administrative physicians now must spend a significant amount of energy reviewing charts that don't initially reflect safe and benchmark care. This is necessary because, as mentioned before, very few "fallouts" may significantly impact national grades, hospital reputations, and governmental penalties and incentives. It also reveals fertile soil for PI (process improvement) activities.

An administrative physician review does help us determine if there is inappropriate care or just insufficient documentation. For example, the timing of treatment in the ED for a patient with sepsis is quite regimented and needs to meet strict time guidelines. Antibiotics must be administered within three hours once the diagnosis of sepsis is considered. Failure to meet this timeline creates what is known as a "fallout." The hospital is graded on the percentage of compliance with this process. This is not an inappropriate measure, as we are committed to early recognition and early antibiotic therapy for severe sepsis. We know that compliance with the sepsis bundle makes a considerable positive impact on the treatment of these patients, including their long-term survival.

Sometimes, the suspicion of severe sepsis is based on just looking at vital signs or preliminary lab tests.

Under some circumstances, low-risk patients may present with suggestive signs/symptoms that automatically get "counted" and therefore start the clock for the onset of treatment. When we analyzed our success rate in compliance with early treatment, we found that a small, but not insignificant, number of patients fell into this category. The remedy for this situation was not directed at clinical improvement but at the need for the treating ED specialist to *document* that the patient "did not have severe sepsis" in the medical record, thereby eliminating it from the sepsis bucket and the count of non-adherence to protocols. Three or four people, including a "sepsis coordinator," were integrated into this process. Although legitimate, this focus on documentation is problematic in terms of where energy is directed in the care of patients.

- We cannot allow the health information system and the secondary information stream to capture the focus of care.

- Recognize that health information systems don't require fewer resources to maximize safety and quality.

- Continue to develop other modes of documentation, including "smart glasses" (93), voice-to-word processing, scribes, etc., to allow for a return to bedside focus.

  o Facebook released Ray-Ban stories in September 2021: glasses with built-in cameras and headphones that let you shoot photos and videos

  o Google Glasses are used in various medical clinic settings with varied results and acceptance.

- Expect that uncertainty, complexity, statistical variability, "unpredictability, hidden interactions and dynamism . . . will cause new risks and dangers not previously anticipated" [(94) Sutcliff p. 216].

- The current state of AI can provide significant input into algorithms and even intuition (pattern recognition & projections). Still, it cannot offer the emotional intelligence necessary for highly adaptable and communicative care.

- AI has significant limitations, and the fact that it requires more resources is also a *substantial barrier to the interaction of staff with patients and with each other.* Even when engaged in direct communication with a patient, clinicians and nurses have the physical computer between them, frequently blocking eye contact and limiting physical contact. The Covid pandemic has only solidified these care trends. Physicians were discouraged from entering patient rooms because of the risk of exposure, particularly at the beginning of the pandemic, because of the limited availability of PPE (personal protective equipment). The medical system in the United States was caught flat-footed when acquiring appropriate PPE. The well-published account of the deadly and demoralizing impact on health care workers in New York during Covid-19 made any exposure to patients very concerning.

Despite becoming very clear that the virus was almost totally spread through airway transmission, the trend to treat all patients without touching and limiting any direct contact has continued. We now have a generation of new clinicians who have learned care and trained in academic centers during the Covid pandemic. For the most part, these young doctors embrace limited direct exposure to patients they care for. This trend can also be appreciated when watching the staff minimally interact with patients while managing the demands of the electronic health record.

The old team was varied and dependent on the patient's situation and comprised multiple members in heavy communication. The new team is the practitioner and the computer, principally responsible for implementing communication.

Years ago, when I was making a site visit to evaluate the efficacy of sepsis care in a busy city emergency department, I noted a patient diagnosed with sepsis that clinically looked very unstable and was "falling off the sepsis cliff." Since I had no authority or medical staff privileges to care for patients at this hospital, I immediately identified the nurse caring for the patient and informed her of my concern. She went directly to her computer station and started typing. I asked what she was doing, and she told me that she was informing the doctor of the change in the patient's status.

The computer had become the primary source of communication even in a dire emergency. Since that time in the ED, we have become more reliant on our computers as an interface to facilitate care. The risk to the functionality of the care team is undeniable, but we are stuck in the mire of systems designed originally to manage the financial aspects of care.

A clinical platform and processes are often missing to identify, communicate, and coordinate all the various aspects and locations of care. Such systems are vital in order to provide a fluid and efficient experience for individualized patient circumstances. Tailored systems now exist that can minimize the workload of identifying patients and issues, provide information to the "doers" in a one-step manner, and disperse appropriate status information to the entire team (as well as track the large data sets for evaluation and educational uses). These systems combine AI, multilevel communication capabilities, and *projections* to maximize resources.

The design of these systems is to assist communication between the team, not replace it with computer-based protocols. This is particularly true when evaluating continuity or *whole patient care*. We are now responsible for the care of patients before they enter the medical system, while they are in the acute hospital phase, and monitoring their progress in the post-acute phase whether they are at home, in a SNIF (Skilled Nursing Facility), or in assisted living, or even when they are labeled as homeless. *A health information system can be the answer for coordinating the various aspects of care by facilitating human contact, not replacing it.*

CULTURE

In the early pages of this work, I discussed the first **W** or **WHAT**. An organization is heavily a reflection of its culture. What are our backbones as we strive for safe care, quality care, and meeting the elements of *quadruple aim*? We have talked a great deal about *bias* as it pertains to decision-making and patient care, but it also plays a significant role in the culture of any organization. Modern health organizations have strived to incorporate essential thinking from engineers and have tried to adopt concepts from the airline and nuclear power industries, particularly when enhancing safety. These are the solid internal structures of the psychology and physiology of high-reliability organizations.

There is no doubt that the size and complexity of major healthcare organizations have morphed from individual doctors' offices and local hospitals into the behemoths that they are today. Engineered solutions fit most well into the matrix of complex organizations and standardization of the operational rule. The goal of perfection and zero harm becomes the primary overlying mandate.

Engineering thinking has suggested that safety and quality in aviation and nuclear power have much to teach the medical arena. Over the last several decades, we have seen applications previously in the purview of airline pilots and military jet jockeys become standard practice for clinicians. This has been a tremendously successful strategy and is the basis of multiple books and papers suggesting that these tools be widely used in the medical arena. Yet, as Dr. Gawande points out in his book Checklist Manifesto [(95) pg 35], "Sick people are tremendously more various than airplanes. In a study of forty-one thousand trauma patients in the state of Pennsylvania-just trauma patients found- that they had 1,224 different injury-related diagnoses in 32,261 unique combinations. That's like having 32,261 kinds of airplanes to land."

In Still Not Safe, Wears and Sutcliff say, "There is a danger that the rhetoric of perfection prevents the important discussion of the realities of everyday clinical work. Given that complex systems have elements of unpredictability, hidden interactions, and dynamism . . . there will always be new risks and dangers not previously anticipated" [(96) p. 216].

Sutcliff and her co-authors and Dr. Gawande are not making excuses for medical errors or poor quality. They merely point out that the statistical formula for calculations must be adjusted to encompass uncertainty, complexity, and variability. The parallel theme is the essential elements of humans taking care of humans. The variability on both sides of the medical equation forces us to look carefully at more than checklists, computer-based alarms and notifications, redundancy, and resources.

As tools to assist clinicians, engineered solutions can literally be life-saving. Electronic health information systems, checklists, compulsory double checks, procedural time-outs, advanced diagnostic technologies and many other mechanical devices (such as end-tidal CO_2 monitors that monitor intubated patients) have had a tremendously powerful positive impact on health care.

- The electronic health record has multiple areas where a clinician cannot move forward without first completing certain information. An example would be the mandatory drop-down about allergies before an antibiotic can be ordered. There may be so many of these checklists on any given patient that moving forward in the patient's care becomes hugely time-sensitive and ungainly.

- Checklists, either computer or paper-based, are standard for many procedures. Most national organizations have accepted this contrivance, but compliance is not total, and avoidable failures are still common.

- Monitor alarms are constantly sounding in the daily operations of an intensive care unit and throughout the other acute care settings. Cardiac monitors, oxygen sensors, intravenous medication applications, and multiple other alarms are constantly in use. Patients often complain about the "noise" that prevents them from getting rest, but a more critical consideration is *alarm fatigue* amongst the staff. There are so many alarms that are frequently either shut off or disregarded.

- Double checks are used in an increasing list of medications. Insulin, for example, must be checked by two RN nurses before administration. This is because these *high-risk meds* have potential and significant safety concerns. Yet the process for the double-check is often quite cursory in terms of drug identification, amount to be administered, route of administration, appropriateness of meds, and even patient identification. The application is too common in the hectic life of acute hospital care for all elements to be followed religiously.

- *Time-outs* are recommended for all procedures and require the entire team, whether in the operating room, the emergency department, or elsewhere. The purpose is for the whole team to have a brief opportunity to validate the correct procedure, location, patient, personnel, and materials. The bottom line is it allegedly forces a pause for *critical thinking*.

- End-tidal CO_2 monitors are relatively simple devices attached to endotracheal tubes after a patient is intubated. They simply turn yellow to assure clinicians that CO_2 from the body is being expelled.

This is a technique to support the appropriate placement of a breathing tube.

- Utilizing the above methodologies supports the engineer's view of culture. There is no doubt that we have moved considerably down the path of safety and quality because of these views. Yet the application and compliance to the types of "tools" elucidated above have not guaranteed an absolutely safe or quality environment. Our culture relies heavily on these engineered marvels and the data from counting the compliance. As we have said, one of the specific reasons that we judge quality and safety on compliance metrics is *that we can*. This data can be derived from multiple sources without ever having to understand the dimensions of the clinical course and its variability and uncertainty.

Turning toward the psychologist's view of our complex medical system reveals their bias regarding the role of human involvement and the human propensity toward *error* and *non-compliance*. Safety scientists agree that most medical errors and noncompliance are not based on a lack of knowledge but on a lack of critical thinking and the time and opportunity to do it. David Marx, who is one of the fathers of today's safety movement, recognizes the failings of humans in the system and believes that the role of the system engineer is to *limit human choices through engineered processes*. He states that "humans are not programmed to follow the rules and that the prescription for error reduction is system redesign" [(97) D. Marx, Cal Poly Lecture].

Although I appreciate the utilization of technology that limits the uncertainty of human behavior, I would like to think that the thirty-five years I spent as an emergency department physician caring for thousands of patients in countless variable circumstances was facilitated by my ability to utilize my human side, that my skill was based on my ability to adjust rapidly, leave behind my biases and those of the operational structure, and make critical decisions in the best interest of the patients. In some cases, even the ability to communicate with patients and my team came not from the structure but from human adaptability.

"Doctor, the patient in bed ten is out of control and won't let us get close to him. I have called security to help hold him down and restrain him."

Grace, the charge nurse, approached me with wide eyes and obvious concern. Her fears were justified as this type of patient could seriously harm themselves, delay care, and subject the staff to unnecessary harm.

"What do we know about him?" I asked.

"He vomited, passed out, after drinking with his buddies for Saint Patrick's Day, but he has a 'heart condition,' according to the paramedics that brought him in."

I cautiously approached and found the patient swinging wildly at the staff, even with the paramedics trying to control him.

"Now, hold on a minute, old son." With my best Irish accent, I said, "Your friends are worried about you and just wanted us to check you out."

He froze and, with effort, focused on me. "You the doc? He asked?"

That was only the beginning of a rather tricky evaluation, but at least it was a start. I projected to him some acceptance of the rules, and he recognized that I was there to help him. All protocols aside, human contact ultimately allowed us to care for him in the safest situation.

Unfortunately, the focus on the data, much of which comes from outside sources, can become an organization's culture. There is a trend in large health care systems expressly to adopt standardized performance measures in response to data streams. There is great value in this, but it cannot replace the commitment and accountability of the staff, nor should it replace local expertise and solutions developed for specific markets and geographies. "One size does not fit all," as the advertisement on the side of a city bus states. This statement was about a popular athletic shoe but had great application to the culture, particularly an organization's "human" culture.

In his book, *The Art of Action* (98), Stephen Bungay understands replacing human values and performance with metrics.

Organizations like processes, but they adore metrics. The knowledge gap acts like a vacuum that sucks metrics in. Their precision creates the satisfying illusion that they lack ambiguity, and our ability to collect and collate them creates an equally seductive feeling of control. Advances in technology have allowed for the collection and dissemination of even more measures. Adoration has turned into infatuation. Infatuation leads to perversity. Metrics become an end unto themselves. This danger is particularly pronounced if the metrics are not simply monitored to see whether things are on track but are turned into targets that define performance and individual success. If they are further linked to compensation, the danger becomes acute. Then, if faced with a choice between optimizing targets and what really matters, people optimize the targets. [(99) Pg 204]

We have spent a fair amount of time discussing particular data streams, more from an opportunity point of view rather than an endpoint. Avoiding the seductiveness of data as an endpoint, how best can we process the now overwhelming stream of information that will define the culture of the organization and help us plan a path of *action*?

For data to have a meaningful path to action, it must follow the following outlined path:

COLLECTION, VALIDATION, PRIORITIZATION, AND ANALYSIS

To facilitate assembly, we have collected national data from CMS (five-star) and private agencies that collate government, hospital and patient surveys, hospital audits, and infectious disease system data. There can be as many as 660 individual data points per month. Now streams of new e-data come directly from documentation in the charts and do not go through the coding and billing inputs. These reports are directly uploaded to the government and do not readily offer an opportunity for validation. The good news is that national data sets are increasingly timely. The bad news is that they may present a skewed picture of actual patient care and operations.

On the basis of numerous attributes described previously, we utilize the Intuitive Opportunity Index to highlight a select few specific data streams and then spend considerable clinical and analytical resources delving into the data. This realistically allows us to understand the clinical and operational data and look for opportunities to improve it. Analysis and direct action are impossible for multiple large data sets without the capability for prioritization. In addition, the biggest challenge, as referenced by Bungay in The Art of Action, is to look at the analytical results and not at the data sets. This sounds obvious, but convincing leadership to find opportunities rather than concentrate on the data is sometimes quite problematic. The focus should be "less on metrics and dashboards which are subject to misinterpretation, effort substitution and gaming" [(100) Sutcliff p. 217–218].

Utilizing the data to make a significant change from the engineer's point of view requires reengineering systems and processes. In the complex, changing world of patient care, this is not easy and is often accompanied by significant pain on the part of the utilizers of the system. A small change in the electronic health record often becomes the fodder for huge discussions at medical staff committee meetings. Physicians often have to alter their standards of operation to meet the needs of the newly "scientifically" derived systems.

↯ Engaging people, nurses, doctors, therapists, social workers, care coordinators, and technicians of all types in process improvement is a difficult task. This cannot be done by fiat, or rather it can be tried this way but often fails. Executives that traditionally make pronouncements, which are then expected to be permeated throughout clinical staff members, sometimes will meet open resistance but more commonly meet silent nonperformance. Bringing an understanding of the issues and the need for process improvement and enlisting the local staff and their identified and non-identified leaders has much more favorable results.

If understanding the science of process improvement through education, understanding, and compliance is complex, the challenge of human behavior is much more so. If the human participant is an overseer, their role may be critical but limited to circumstances with an unusual deviation from the norm. In medicine, the human being is central to the operational formula and is often faced with wildly different situations from the norm: complex, uncertain, and time-sensitive. In addition, slight deviations could have immediate and long-term severe consequences. This is the challenge of critical thinking as a core competency and why system engineers try to factor it out of performance equations.

In his book Human Error, James Reason sets the stage for the frailties of critical thinking, particularly during time-sensitive acute, urgent, or emergent situations. Studies in the 1970s from advanced continuous-process industries indicated that "for the most part, they (operators) were applying short sequences of heuristics, or diagnostic rules of thumb" [(101) p. 241]. Heuristics are often biased by experience and focus on the most recent information rather than on a comprehensive review. Perhaps this is why some of our most seasoned professionals can make mistakes or errors of omission.

Reason then explains some of the other compensatory functions that impact critical decision-making.

- Attention is only directed at a very small part of the total problem space at any one time.

- There is a selection of direct attention to "logically" essential aspects of the problem space.

- There is a tendency to apply familiar but inappropriate solutions.

- The influence of availability bias has the tendency to prefer diagnosis and strategies that spring readily to mind.

Rote decisions based on standard Process, Procedure, or Protocol can be done if everyone "follows the rules." Errors of omission can be reduced by alarms, checklists, double checks, and constant supervision. This is difficult in the hectic health care environment but has proven to minimize errors and improve quality. Controlling human behavior and the application of critical thinking are the challenges moving forward.

An executive cannot be successful if their approach is "I say; you do." Successful organizations spend a lot of time and resources to ensure that their people have the "right stuff" to succeed. Indeed, as discussed, this means the correct organizational framework and the tools necessary to do the job correctly. Still, it ultimately comes down to the people in human business-like medicine. In The Art of Action [(102) p. 229], Bungay describes elements of a Leadership *Trinity* that are demonstrated in successful organizations of all types.

✓   Directing: This is made up of intellectual elements that focus on developing strategy, giving direction and building organizations. This part of the Trinity has the authority, responsibility and duty of direction.

✓   Leading: This is made up of human and moral attributes and focuses on Task, Team and individuals.

✓   Managing: This is the most technical aspect and is focused on resourcing, managing and organizing.

Bungay's characterization of the Leadership Trinity helps us distinguish the elements of leadership and management within the larger role necessary for organizational success. The focus on Team and Individuals echoes our discussion on prioritizing the *balance* between our human elements, and the technological advances that we currently see in our daily lives.

In the earlier pages of the book, I spent a considerable amount of time characterizing the culture necessary for long-term success in a hospital setting. A good part of that success comes from a leadership structure that can communicate directly and indirectly the inherent goals of the organization. Leaders must be able to reach people at a midbrain level and convey the feelings and the ownership of the myriad of daily tasks in a complicated health care system. In their book *Extreme Ownership* (103), Jocko Willink and Leif Babin describe in great detail the demands of a SEAL team leader and the ultimate responsibility one needs to take.

The book takes us through some of the excruciating painful experiences the SEAL teams endured in combat. The message was, that the leaders had to own and take responsibility for their actions, subordinates, and the team. While nearly not as graphic, the parallels to the acute care hospital are quite accurate. The rapidly evolving issues, complexities, and uncertainties create a significant risk.

In the case of the hospital, the risk flows primarily to the patients, but as demonstrated during Covid, the risk is quite genuine for the staff as well, not only in the real risk of contagion but also in the emotional toll that the pandemic has inflicted. Reading about the experiences of our soldiers in the Middle East, one additional theme becomes very apparent. No matter at what level of leadership or command we find the decision-maker, *trust* is the essential quality. "I have got your back" echoes implicitly in the culture of a successful hospital or military environment. The staff looks at executive leadership to provide an environment that supports their capabilities, and the executives look at the staff to be accountable for their performance. The other parallel is that unexpected death is a constant in war and the hospital and demands our full engagement.

Looking at the positions that are titled in a health care organization, we would be able to identify a series of leaders. Like the military, the hospital organization encompasses many layers of leadership.

Both Sinek in his book <u>Leaders Eat Last</u> (104) and Willink in <u>Extreme Ownership</u> (105) are not bashful about enumerating leadership responsibilities and the ownership that comes with the title or rank. SEAL teams have unique attributes that downplay the hierarchy and make every team member responsible for the team and themselves.

✶ It is easy to comprehend how the SEAL team becomes a band of brothers in war. This may not be as obvious in a hospital or other medical setting, but ask almost any staff member how they made it through a difficult shift, and they will point to their peers. "Our intelligence gives us ideas and instructions. But it is our ability to cooperate that actually helps us get things done.' [(106) Pg. 95] Sinek goes on to say, "Trust and commitment are feelings that we get from the release of chemical incentives deep in our Limbic brain.". It is this feeling permeating all levels of Leadership and Team that makes the human-to-human context of medical care absolutely necessary.

The use of the computer for communication between all staff members has unfortunately gone far to isolate, dehumanize, and undermine the team and the connection to our patients.

We tend to look past the notion of good leaders and prioritize good managers. "Good management means making the maximum use of resources, including money and people. Leading is a human activity that is moral and emotional. The work of a leader is to motivate and, if possible, inspire follow-ers . . . Leaders have to balance their attention between defining and achiev-ing specific tasks, building and maintaining the team as a team, and meeting the needs of and developing the individuals within it" [(107) Bungay p. 229].

⟨ Nothing in the rule book says one cannot be a good leader and a good manager. I worked in a health care system that combined with another system to achieve the massive value of scale. Although this might have made good sense in maximizing the benefits of corporate medicine, it had a significant impact on leadership. Local leadership became management and deferred to leaders at the corporate level. Underscoring that leadership depends on human moral and emotional activity, the gap between local management and corporate leaders can devalue the human connections that provide the essence of ownership, accountability, and caring.

Transforming local leaders into managers effectively undermined their "leaning in" at a midbrain level and their ability to reach their staff, make effective decisions, and motivate action at the local level.

The reliance on the computer, overwhelming data, minimizing direct contact with patients and teammates, corporate medicine making decisions for hundreds of hospitals rather than individual hospitals, and large-scale standardization undermine the ownership that leaders throughout the organization must embrace.

The Rx

Significant parts of this book have been focused on where medicine is today. We have looked at the first **WHAT** and described the current culture, leadership, and tools that define our organization. The majority of discussion does come from looking at the modern medical workplace, but by inference, it is also a peek at all companies and organizations.

In hospitals specifically, human assets are the most valuable and costly element, and therefore we have looked at **WHY** we are here and our psychological drive. We have looked at those factors that impact the **WHY**, the tools we use in our job, and the factors that affect our decisions. Our feelings, biases, the impact of emotional intelligence and intuition, our interdependence on our peers, and our connection to our patients have been presented.

I realize that many organizations stand on the threshold of changing how they serve their goals. Technical advances continue to erode the role of people in their businesses. Machines may do it better, more economically, and faster in many industries, but the *product* in medicine remains the health and welfare of our patients. Technology must be directed at allowing us to do this better, not try to re-engineer humans out of the delivery system.

The third **W**, **WHAT**, is very technical, and I apologize. Still, it is crucial to understand the methodology and results of how we, like medical facilities and professionals, are delivering the health care product. Internal and external data is a tremendous motivator for improvement. We spent many years justifying and explaining our errors and inefficiencies because validated, timely, and statistically, significant information was unavailable. That information is increasingly concurrent and comparable on a national level. It now serves as signposts for improvement in safety and quality activities in most hospitals, clinics, and organizations.

The fourth **W**, **WHY**, analyzes and puts the information to use. The organizational tools exist to ask the correct questions. Our quest is to prioritize the resulting data into an improvement culture that can continue to reduce error and improve quality. Improvements start when we understand **WHY** stuff happens or doesn't happen, rather than reacting to a number or statistic.

The final **W**, which I guess could stand for **WHEW**, finally represents what we are going to do about it.

The prescription for the future of health care is not a single "wonder drug" but consists of multiple considerations that crisscross, overlap, and even confront each other. However, these considerations are not limited to medical facilities but are appropriate in any organization where people are recognized as the most valuable resource.

✓ As part of the first **W**, *culture needs to be the first topic* because it consists of so many forces and influences that it encompasses all the other attributes of organizational success.

CULTURE

Working in an organization, large or small, demands an understanding of the culture, an appreciation of it, and the need to become part of it. A health care organization that depends on its human resources must have some level of overarching limbic or emotional connection. The work of medicine itself mainly provides a good part of this. When all is said and done, most of us understand that our business is humans taking care of humans, which helps define **WHY** we as individuals are here.

✦ Our culture is rapidly changing around us. In the supermarket, self-checkout utilizing scanners makes the process faster, allowing for concurrent inventory and utilization data. After the initial setup, it seriously impacts salaries and personnel. The pandemic has also changed where we work. Remote work is so omnipresent, that it has now become the study of academicians and is regularly taught in MBA programs (108). WFH (work from home) will continue unabated even when Covid becomes endemic, and the best guess is it will become some hybridized model. The pressure on the culture of all organizations and the mores of the next generation will be significantly impacted by these forces. Ultimately how industries such as health care will adapt will test our resolve or even our need to rely on humans as our principal resource.

Successful organizations in the past have defined elements of culture as essential in succeeding, and although there may be differences, there are common themes. In his textbook <u>Organizational Culture and Leadership</u> [(109) p. 3-5], Edgar Shein characterizes the observational elements of culture.

Shein's concepts as applied to the hospital environment:

- **"Observed behavioral regularities when people interact"**:

- Walking through the medical-surgical floor of a hospital and observing the dozens of people working there, one will note the constant hum of verbal interaction. This is still true even though so much time is spent servicing the needs of the computerized health record. Facial expressions and random brief utterances are often the keys to understanding the mood and stresses of acute patient care. This validates that we "are all in the same boat" but expresses the need for cooperation, collaboration, and understanding, which is necessary daily.

  o These activities also help define the mores of the organization. They may be so strong that different units (Med Surg vs ICU) within the hospital have different languages and acceptable personal habits.

    o   These "baseline" interactions are critical and cannot be replaced with technological substitutes.

- **"Climate"**:

- The physical layout of a hospital helps conveys the feeling of comfort and caring. Patient private rooms, for example vs Rooms with 2 to 3 patients permit a different hospital experience.

    o   The Covid pandemic has reaffirmed that the physical climate must project a feeling of safety for both patients and staff. This does not mean just the presence of isolation rooms and the compulsive use of PPE, but the respect shown by the staff for the individual patient and their needs.

- **"Formal rituals and celebrations"**:

- Publicly announced principles and celebrations of publicized national safety and quality scores reinforce the public perception of hospital quality.

    o   Additional honors such as the Daisy Award for excellence in nursing, promoted by a "pinning ceremony", promote comradery and self-pride within the staff.

- **"Formal philosophy"**:

    o   Broad policies and ideologic principles may appear as highlighted signs and banners in hospital corridors, brochures, and company letterheads.

- **"Rules of the game"**:

- Knowing the ropes and being taught those standards by existing team members. This is considerably easier in small- to medium-sized facilities, where new additions are embraced and become members of the "family."

- **"Identity and image of self":**

    o   The wearing of color-coded team scrubs has helped patients identify the role of individual staff members, but it has also supported the staff's unique identity and sense of belonging.

✓ Certainly, Shein's description classically helps define our culture. Still, there must be a significant sea change spurred on by the generational change of the millenniums and the recent pressure of Covid-19 on organizations.

- Culture can't be static, as it is the foundation of our ability to adopt, adapt, and change to the uncertainty, complexity, and even confusion of our current times. The ability to be successful comes from reacting to what is happening, not what we think should be happening. The organization must be limber enough to quickly respond to change, understand the need to evaluate quickly, analyze data and trends, and prioritize responses. This is certainly not easy, particularly in a field as highly regulated as health care and impacted by outside forces such as unionization.

- It is essential to integrate generational changes into organizational culture. The conversion of the hospital and hospital systems into *health care systems* requires incorporating *pre- and post-acute services.*

- The recognition of the need for care across the continuum has significantly altered the landscape, putting enormous demands on hospitals, clinics, providers, payors, and patients.

- Conversion to WPC (*whole patient care*) was attempted approximately twenty-five to thirty years ago in the United States, with limited success. (except for Kaiser Permanente, which focused on the blue color working class of patients and contracting directly with employers).

- The old rules are changing, and reluctantly in some cases, even the formal articulated philosophies have had to be replaced by more fluid and responsive rhetoric as well.

- On the ground, decisions and *local authority* are intrinsic to reacting and controlling the high degree of variability within organizations, particularly in large and national ones. A centralized standardized decision-making process has severe limitations in adapting to local cultures, local needs, and local mores.

- The penetration of the computer-based care system and the need for continuity across a much larger canvas have exacerbated the need for processes and new tools that allow for integration, collaboration, and accountability. These tools are now available, but there is reluctance and difficulty in integrating them into large highly structured corporate health information systems.

- The modern health care structure must include a more advanced and integrated system for patient inclusion in information, decision making, and responsibility. Maintenance of normal blood pressures in risk populations, for example, cannot be only on the shoulders of the provider and his/her medical and nutritional armamentarium but must incorporate the patient with a very high level of accountability.

- Home Health monitoring is a step toward placing better knowledge and control in the hands of patients with appropriate supervision.

Shein's classic description of *culture* gets us to a jumping-off place to ask the question, "What should it look like?" in response to our current situation. Culture is the most critical element in articulating a *common goal*, and a common goal is an essential factor in defining culture. An organization cannot be run by defining aspects of care in hospitals solely by proclamation. Roughly translated, task definition, job description, or policies and procedures cannot replace *ownership* (in Willink's terms), accountability, and commitment at every position.

Maintaining a *midbrain level connection* to the job takes work on everyone's part. Scientific design of the workplace, tools, and processes has gone a long way at improving quality and safety but, in some ways, has undermined the organizational commitment toward *humans taking care of humans.*

An indication of ownership is the distinction in an ordinary nursing conversation heard on the medical/surgical floor.

"Can you please help me turn the patient in Room 204?"

vs

"Can you please help me turn *my* patient in Room 204?"

Changing one word reflects ownership and accountability that reflects the midbrain connection to what we do and transcends relying on technology or standardized procedures.

Increasingly, there is a tendency for the bedside caregiver to *take for granted* that the scientifically designed process will eliminate safety risks and noncompliance with benchmarked quality actions. The *process design* approach has been highly successful in aviation and nuclear power. Still, it is somewhat more problematic in medicine, where uncertainty, complexity, and deviations from the norm are the rule. It does, however, raise the issue of *human error*, which can only be partly mitigated by scientific process design and is inherent with human-based resources.

The more humans and the more interactions, the more possibility there is for human error to occur. Eliminating error through process design, redundancy, standardization, and technology has been very effective. Nuclear power and aviation have come dramatically close to eliminating the possibility of error. In medicine, the proportion of decisions and consequent actions continue to be impacted by patients and their complexity. In addition, staff variability, diagnostic uncertainty, and the basic human psyche play a significant role *Critical thinking* remains an essential element in the basis for safe and quality patient care.

✳ Health care systems must move toward truthfully defining and articulating *organizational goals*. If you ask most folks working in health care, they say that financial goals are the tail wagging the dog. Of course, financial success, or at least stability, is a significant factor or goal for all organizations. However, it cannot achieve workplace satisfaction on a deep psychological level, particularly with the current primary healthcare factors.

For example, LOS (length *of stay*) is a significant discussion point on daily rounds, stressing the financial implications of extra days or, even worse, uncompensated days. The discussion should instead focus on the opportunities that this metric presents. It is only one measure of understanding the

✳ efficiency of patient care, which is an important *quality* issue. The appropriate LOS of a patient depends not only on their progression through disease or response to medication or procedures, but also on opportunities to look at how we have managed their overall care and prepared them for *discharge*.

✳ I find even the term "discharge" unsettling. I think it reflects the relinquishment of responsibilities for the patient, which is not correct. When patients leave the acute care setting, they are rarely ready to resume normal activities. Patients are better, not well, when they leave the acute care setting in today's world. There is a definite need for continued services, even physical placement, in some circumstances. There is always a need for continued care, even if supplied by the patient or the family. I have tried to change the vocabulary of hospital discharge to *"transfer"* or *"move to another level of care,"* which I believe better reflects the needs of the continuum.

This process, at first glance, does not seem applicable to other industries, but reaching out to their customers following purchases for help or problems has a proven track record of enhancing customer loyalty. A follow-up phone call after the patient leaves the acute setting is a valuable tool in the medical realm. It helps the *patient satisfaction score*, and it helps to minimize post-acute problems, solve issues, and reduce readmissions.

The tools for getting patients out of the hospital don't always seem to be aligned with taking the best care of patients. When looking at LOS from a patient and hospital perspective, it is easy to oversimplify it simply as a measure of efficiency. LOS does have a significant psychological impact on our caregivers. We lose a great deal if the caregiver is primarily judged by complying with standards and numerical values (like a LOS of 3.7 days). They should be focusing on the *human goal* of the best care for the patient and *feeling good* about what they do. An emotional sense of their interactions, communication, problem-solving, and empathy with patients is realistically one of the critical elements of job satisfaction. *Our job as leaders is to ensure that this connection is not lost.*

The issue of LOS must also be put in perspective of the need for *continuity of care.* As discussed on multiple pages in this work, continuity of patient care requires significant additional resources in what is now a fragmented system. For the most part, these other resources to ensure continuity have not been traditionally necessary and are not without significant cost. The demand for additional resources does not have an evident direct positive impact on the bottom line or return on investment. The *extra* case manager or care coordinator to provide coordination across the medical continuum is an expense that is not easy to justify merely based on *good care.*

Surprisingly, it has not been easy to justify even when data shows that good care also means fewer readmissions to the hospital, better patient satisfaction scores, and less demand on the health care system in general. Many companies outside the medical field have developed considerable resources to manage unsatisfied customers. This pays significant dividends and enhances customer loyalty. Post-hospital discharge phone calls have been shown to reduce readmissions, improve long-term outlook, and positively impact patient loyalty.

Following culture with well-accepted *goals* that transcend all levels of staff, we have focused on leadership as a key to organizational success. Leaders are often characterized by folks living in the C-suite. They have titles, executive assistants, catered lunches brought to their offices, and limited openings in their schedules. Leadership is also endowed and visible at multiple levels in an acute care hospital, including the bedside staff. The personal acceptance of this role as a leader starts to differentiate staff from those trying to follow the rules and those engaged in critical thinking. This thinking is hooked to an emotional attachment to the work; the patient is always in the crosshairs and staff ownership and accountability are inherent in everything they do.

✷ Accepting a leadership role, the title of a position notwithstanding is expected in the acute hospital setting. There are too many nooks and crannies, too many essential departments, and too many job silos to function without local commitment and leadership. Quick reactions and decision-making demand leadership at every level that only ownership can provide. This concept transcends the walls of medicine and is integral in many businesses where human resources play a critical role.

Facilitating the critical integration of human resources into the hospital world, but even in other fields not as floridly dependent on people, requires an understanding and management philosophy.

✓ The mnemonic for this management philosophy is the *vowels: A, E, I, O, U.*

- **A: Awareness/Action**

- **E: Engage/Empower**

- **I: Individual/ Integration**

- **O: Ownership**

- **U: Understanding/Unexpected/Unbalanced**

Awareness

In a highly educated professional environment, awareness is assumed, but there are significant gaps, unfortunately. It is not always effective if the presumption is that awareness about current processes and behaviors, data, and operational issues is passed down from executive leadership and incorporated into everyday life. Despite emails, meetings, and conferences, there is always material that leadership is unaware of or too busy to deal with, particularly from the patient bedside level. This is not atypical in any organization. In addition, even important critical information is usually passed down through multiple levels of leadership and management before there is a credible opportunity for staff to become aware of it. Everything from significant policy changes to patient care data may be true.

The mechanisms for this level of communication bump into the dynamics of a busy acute care facility and associated post-acute services. Too many moving parts: differential shift times, a conglomeration of different units with slightly different cultures, uncontrollable critical care demands, and outside forces and pressure are typical hurdles. Hospitals and other essential services like police and fire function on a 24/7 schedule that requires a command structure accommodating for the diffusion of leadership and authority.

Some executive leaders are better at this than others. This depends on their relationships, communication style and skills, and the inherent difficulty of reaching multiple levels of staff. Middle management often tries to fill in the gaps, but they run into the same dilemmas. Communication of serious import cannot simply be shared by posters, emails, and logs. They are open to translation and do not carry any emotional force behind them. Person-to-person communication through team meetings is a much more realistic approach. Still, it is seriously curtailed by the immediate needs of patients and to some degree by the need to limit dedicating resources to nonclinical activities.

Identifying local leadership, and empowering them to communicate personally with staff, supported by executive and management leadership, can provide awareness and support individual education and acceptance. This is not "They want us to do this," but "Why we do this" and what it means to the ultimate patient care goal.

We have achieved significant success by identifying stakeholders and local leaders to deal with safety or quality issues. They live the specifics every day.

They know their teams' strengths and weaknesses. They have the best insight into the vicissitudes of their work environment and have the most emotional (midbrain) investment. Reinforcement from "up the chain of command" is essential but is not the backbone of this process. In the medical field, this is often referred to as caring, the definition of which is ownership, accountability, and commitment.

As we have seen, copious information from government and national sources exists. In addition, currently, hospitals and hospital systems provide an increasingly current amount of data, often monthly, on operations and process compliance. This information may even be used to adjudicate financial bonuses amongst the management staff.

Even with an analysis that approaches the answer to **WHY** it happens, published data cannot be expected to facilitate improvement unless it is specifically directed and embraced. The rate of elective C-sections in obstetrics, for example, may be of interest to management across all service lines in a hospital. However, the information must be personalized enough to galvanize action amongst the obstetricians, the nurses, and the midwives that ultimately determine the timing and selection of care. This sometimes requires the tedious process of individual patient reviews by a team of professionals. These sessions, protected by confidentiality, can get quite organic, but the dialogue stays within the family and can significantly improve all aspects of patient care.

Awareness may be the first step toward action, but we cannot assume that there is cause and effect. Validated, pertinent local data must be *prioritized* to help stimulate action. We are all too busy to have a midbrain attachment to the hundreds of metrics now available monthly. Using the IOI (intuitive opportunity index) can help choose meaningful data sets with high potential financial, quality, and safety impact. Local leaders and staff must understand the direct benefit of a specific "measure" in their everyday life at a gut level.

Of all the considerations of the reams of data available, the most crucial consideration is how to initially *prioritize* and then utilize the information in an impactful manner. The *IOI* gets us partway there, but interaction with the clinicians and what is most important in the patient's direct care should be prioritized.

Currently, items on dashboards all have equal weight for scoring. *Outcome data*, which is recognized as the "gold standard," is complex and based on multiple independent factors and, therefore, is much more challenging to impact psychologically. It doesn't galvanize action in the same manner as it does work on a process measure. These measures are much more in the control of the on-scene clinical operators.

Feeling overwhelmed by the task of reducing pneumonia mortality because of multiple variables may be tackled by focusing on a single operational process, such as the choice and timing of antibiotics.

The staff must additionally understand the **WHY**. It must also be able to internalize the ultimate *goal* of a measure rather than just focusing on compliance with *tools* or processes. In the craziness of hospital life, compliance with wristband scanning to avoid medication errors must have an emotional connection to not hurting a patient. Giving the wrong patient medication proscribed for another individual or mixing up medication can be disastrous to both the patient and the staff. By combining the appropriate engineered design structure to minimize human error or lack of compliance with highly engaged staff with an emotionally vested interest, we have a real shot at reducing error and improving quality.

At one facility, I had the privilege of making individual rounds with the nursing staff. Clinical rounds, in general, are a fantastic time to enhance communication and share information with the many members of the team. In a teaching or quaternary care facility, the primary goal of rounds is to teach medical students and residents (house staff) wisdom from the attending (instructors and professors) staff. In the teaching/learning environment, the subjects of rounds on specific patients may include advances in care, notations from published literature about current best practices, and insights into the decision process about care plans. The "at the bedside" approach has been a standard methodology, is time intensive, and is resourced accordingly.

✻   In a non-teaching facility that takes care of a full spectrum of sick and critically ill patients, rounds provide an opportunity for team involvement and building and are a critical element in situational awareness. They provide a level of insight unavailable from the electronic health record. In addition, they enhance the team approach and are an excellent mechanism for empowering the nursing staff and recognizing the other members of the unit.

✻   In addition to participating in team rounds, I had the opportunity to round with individual nurses on multiple units on a regular weekly basis. The goal was to educate them about the specific disease entities and treatments that their patients represented. This was pretty didactic, but the nurses appreciated the discussion and education. They often did not receive it from hospitalists or other attending physicians because of the time crunch that demanded their attention. I discovered almost universally that the nursing staff, particularly the less experienced ones, were focused on *tasks* and *tools*.

I don't know why I was surprised, as the entire medical complex, even our data, grades, and reputation, hung primarily on our success with tasks and tools. The nursing staff was my last great hope that the requirements to be at the bedside would encourage a different relationship. I would ask the nurse **WHAT** they were doing with a patient and would receive a litany of concrete answers. "I started the IV, gave antibiotics and fluids, then I bath-roomed the patient, redressed the wound, and then I did my nursing notes in the electron health record."

✻   From early on in their education, nurses were focused on the tasks, their importance and the need for best practice, and compliance. This focus was not wrong in satisfying the immediate need for patient care. However, it falls short in understanding the consequences of what they did and even less in understanding the **WHY** of their actions. Part of these "teaching rounds" was an opportunity to discuss the pathophysiology of a patient's illness and why specific tasks had an impact. The nurse's immediate reaction was very positive, as the physical work was put into context.

A more complex proposition for these rounds was changing the conversation to understand the *goals* of care. The nurses, and the staff in general, needed to make an effort to understand the individual patient, their specific needs, and the enormous scope of their care. This included the alternatives the patient needed to consider in the hospital setting and how their decisions impacted the post-acute phase and beyond. These considerations led to better care across the continuum, a thirst for knowledge of quality data relative to the patient, and an increased feeling of *ownership*.

"Doctor, can I ask you a question about *my* patient?" Nina, the nurse, said.

> The doctor, rushing out of the room, replied, "Sure. I'm just about to see a patient in the emergency department, but what do you need?"
>
> Nina walked with the doctor as he was leaving the room. "When will he be discharged, and where is he going?"
>
> "Probably a couple of more days, then he can go home," the doctor said.
>
> "Doctor, he can't even stand by himself right now, so can we consider sending him to acute rehab rather than home if our goal is making him as independent as possible?"
>
> "The family wants him home."
>
> "I understand, but I think they would be open to a short stay in rehab if they want him to be walking and taking care of himself at some level."
>
> "Thanks," the doctor said. "I'll discuss it with the family."

In this situation, the doctor focused on the length of time the patient had received antibiotics, the fact that he remained afebrile, and his laboratory tests showed continued improvement. Because it was "her patient," the nurse was able to step away from tasks and tests and help focus on the goal of patient care across the continuum.

Engage and Empower

"Engagement" in the dictionary is defined as "involve, occupy, engross, absorb, take part, participate, undertake, enter into, etc." Engagement is a two-way street. "Executives can explain to people what they have to achieve and why making them ready to act. By mastering management, they can put people into a position in which they can act. And by leading them effectively, they can sustain people's willingness to carry on until the job is done" [(110) Bungay p. 232].

One of the absolute necessities to ensure engagement is *trust*. The leaders at the top of the pyramid must not only trust their subordinate managers and leaders, but they must demonstrate this trust by allowing for independent action. Without this trust, local leaders of all persuasions will fall back on being followers and refuse accountability for their actions. "I was instructed to do it this way" is not a refrain reflecting long-term passion and commitment.

Realistically, it is not expected that every staff member is fully engaged, but even when it is limited to key individuals, the staff and the patients can feel it. These folks at work are smiling, and although working hard under the most challenging circumstances, they deal with stress most effectively. They understand their jobs and responsibilities but emotionally recognize their accomplishment and the importance of their lives. Part of the distinction is that these individuals have a deep understanding of the second **W** in our cascade. They understand **WHY** they are here. However, even the most balanced, mature individuals need support and validation to help them effectively manage the stress from their uncertain environments. This cannot be accomplished simply by a paycheck or a superior's standard card or letter. The individuals need to recognize how they fit in an organization on an emotional and intellectual level. This needs to be supported enthusiastically by *leadership*.

Bungay defines what he refers to as the *executive trinity*. [(111) 227-232]

1. Command. "An external party grants this, and the commander remains accountable for direction, decision making, and control."

2. Management. "Means making the maximum use of resources, including money and people."

3. Leadership. "[It] is a human activity that is moral and emotional. The leader's work is to motivate and, if possible, inspire followers. Leaders have to balance their attention between defining and achieving the specific task, building and maintaining the team as a team and meeting the needs of the developing individuals within it" [(112) Bungay p. 227–229].

Bugay concludes that "we need less management and more leadership," whether at the executive level or in the daily functions and modeling at the staff level.

A. The task of leadership is to empower the "doers" in the organization.

B. Although there are many forces and pressures on the leaders, they must faithfully represent and be accountable for the organization's goals.

C. . Hospital leadership must genuinely represent the needs of the community and the medical staff and not simply bow to the dictates of the corporate executives.

D. . Leaders must ensure that the staff functionally taking care of patients understand their roles and are accountable for their actions.

Individual

Despite ideally being a part of a highly functional team and the interdependence of the members, we come to work with our own needs and biases. According to David Marx, part of our repertoire as humans is "as we navigate life, we like to collect things, and we will protect those things as property interests" (113). During the lecture, Marx, widely recognized as the founder of Just Culture, enumerated the following human needs and wants.

- Knowledge and skill

- Wealth and tangibles

- Fitness and beauty

- Reputation and acceptance

- Order and stability

- Power and influence

- Independence and autonomy

- Interdependence and belonging

- Fairness and justice

Part of our job as human leaders is the understanding of ourselves as individuals, our needs, and our biases as we deal with the command structure, our associates, teammates, subordinates, and customers. The job cannot define us, but who we are can determine the job. This is probably true of many industries, but it is undoubtedly true in medicine. As humans, our interactions allow us to feel and have emotional connections to what we are doing. *This sharpens focus, enhances commitment and caring, and leads to security and job satisfaction.* It multiplies the importance of everything we do. Administering a medication becomes a step-by-step reflection of our involvement, in addition to just following the path proscribed by engineers and human factor scientists.

We have talked a lot about the impact of *bias* on the kinds of decisions we make and the reactions we have to situations and even colleagues and patients. Perhaps even more important is what we think about ourselves. How much have we internalized the messaging of family and friends over the years? How often have we repeated self-refrains that focus on our strengths and, even more probably, our weaknesses? What we bring to the table reflects who set the table and the elements upon it.

Tom Heller was a sixty-year-old banker and pillar of his community. He could always be found at fundraising and community events. At 3:00 a.m., the paramedics brought him to the emergency department. His wife, who followed the ambulance to the hospital, stated that he had flu-like symptoms for several days, enough that he unusually stayed home from work. He had a persistent fever, poor appetite, and no energy, and he spent two days mostly in bed. As the winter flu was around, the wife did not become overly concerned since Tom was generally in good health without risk factors. She had been awakened at 2:15 a.m. when she heard guttural sounds coming from their bathroom. When she rushed into the bathroom, she found Tom unconscious, unresponsive, and having trouble breathing, so she quickly dialed 911.

On arrival to the ED, Tom was still unresponsive, had extremely low blood pressure, and because of his inability to oxygenate and protect his airway, he was endotracheally intubated. This is an emergency process requiring a team to position the patient, give medications, visualize the vocal cords, and pass an endotracheal tube into the correct position in the trachea to take over the work of breathing for a patient. There was a coordinated but frantic ballet of physicians, nurses, EMTs, respiratory therapists, and radiology techs to ensure the proper placement and positioning of the ET tube. In the ED, the diagnosis of septic shock was made, and he was aggressively treated with fluids and antibiotics.

Patients presenting like Tom with overwhelming sepsis have a very guarded prognosis. He remained in critical condition on the ventilator for days and days. Despite laboratory evidence that his infection was under control, his body had not yet overcome the overwhelming trauma from his illness. Under intensive therapy and observation, he continued in a very unresponsive state. Clarissa, one of the senior nurses taking care of him, developed a relationship with his wife, who was in daily attendance at Tom's bedside. "What kind of things does he like and do together with you?" Clarissa asked. "We love music and like to dance together," his wife replied. The next day Clarissa had Tom sitting up in bed while still on the ventilator, music blaring, and she held his arms out rhythmically, "dancing," as could only happen in an ICU. Tom's eyes fluttered, and that day marked the beginning of his eventual remarkable recovery. Tom remembered none of this, but his wife, who watched Clarissa dance with her husband, has told the tale many times with tears in her eyes.

Clarissa understood on an emotional, intuitive level what Tom needed to kick start his recovery. This was not only providing her patient with excellent care, but she was totally engaged as an individual with his recovery. Bias is not always a bad thing. Approaching a clinical situation with an understanding of one's own humanity and how it translates from early experiences in life is an advantage for a nurse. The qualifier is knowing oneself and accepting biases and how they can be beneficial, as in Clarissa's case. However, as discussed earlier, bias can also confuse appropriate decision-making and even observation.

"The most pervasive obstacle to good thinking is confirmational bias, which refers to the human tendency to search only for evidence that confirms our preferred beliefs . . . The most reliable cure for confirmational bias is interaction with people who don't share your beliefs" (114). Clarissa was not only an excellent nurse but an integral element of a team, where face-to-face communication was the key to care. She also demonstrated "out of the box" thinking, which was encouraged and supported by her ICU colleagues.

As we reflect on our current pandemic, we see so much evidence of the *stress* on our system and all of us trying to survive both psychologically and actually. Many of us have demonstrated significant stress reactions to the demands and situations we have been asked to work. A cottage industry of employee assistance has blossomed owing to the responses to the stress of personal fear, uncertainty, and depression. The pandemic has outlasted the normal favorable stress response. Although an inherent commonality in our field, death and dying have morphed into a dreaded specter in patients, and we could only, at best, support, not cure.

⚥ ⚥ In his book <u>Stress for Success</u> (115), James Loehr offers a program, developed initially for athletes, to train oneself to see stress as an opportunity for success rather than a negative. He distinguishes our capacity from a perspective that exposes the "difference between stress exposure and stress response" [(116) Loehr p. 4]. It is clear from watching the varied stress reactions from the hospital and health care staff to Covid-19 that some of us are better prepared to handle stress, but certain individuals can actually thrive in the environment. Loehr says, "The ultimate impact of stress in your life is determined not by the stress exposure itself but by your response to that exposure."

Loehr describes the ideal state of balance necessary to handle stress, particularly that coming from the chronicity of Covid and some of the hopelessness it spawns. He describes finding "the ideal relationship between stress and recovery . . . and by not changing the mechanics or techniques, but rather by changing what they think and feel."

⚥ Loehr describes the physiology of stress as dopamine and norepinephrine mediated through alpha receptors. These receptors are also impacted by serotonin, which may act to mediate a response. There are then four significant pathways that a stress reaction may take. Adapted from <u>Stress for Success</u>. (117)

1. Immediate fight or flight, leading to a rapid short-term response. If the action is not effective or maintained, it can lead to an intellectual and emotional hyper reaction, which ultimately can produce anxiety or an ulcer.

2. High-intensity passionate productive response. This is fine-tuned, focused, and timely. This response leads to rapid recovery from stress.

3. Intense stressful stimuli that are ignored or not acted upon. This is followed by increasing levels of hormones, which ultimately leads to receptors becoming immune.

4. Intense stimuli that are ignored and become chronic or unrelenting. This leads to insensitivity to the triggers but not the stress it causes.

Points 1, 3, and 4 ultimately lead to helplessness, depression, inactivity disease, and even autoimmune changes.

↝ Loehr suggests that the approach to stress, of trying to avoid it or reduce it, will ultimately fail. Stress, particularly in medicine, and certainly during times such as the current pandemic, is always with us, and we must train our physical, intellectual, and emotional responses. He puts forth a comprehensive training program, but at its heart, it focuses on what we know about ourselves.

↝ "Openly and honestly confront the weaknesses you are targeting for change. Facing the truth about your insecurities, fears, defensiveness, negativism, or lack of discipline anchors you to the real world and sets the record straight." [(118) pg. 56]

We cannot eliminate stress from our daily lives any more than we can ignore our biases. Still, by understanding ourselves, we can maximize our decision-making, critical thinking, and the effectiveness of our lives. Like most personal therapy programs, this skill set takes time, resources, and commitment.

We recognize the absolute need for a long-term strategy to handle the stress of everyday demands, uncertainty, and complexity and to appreciate the unique pandemic experience. The departure of so many health care professionals in the face of the pandemic underscores the need for a highly aggressive program, not just to patch up feelings, but one that is scientifically supported. To realize the significant impact of emotional and hormonal responses, programs must be resourced to facilitate staff to prepare better and adjust to stress.

↝ Throughout the pages of this book, *Team* has been referred to in different manners. It is a social construct. It is a communication device. It is a mechanism for support and recognition. It is an avenue to encourage growth and development, and it is often a key element in the development of individual loyalty. In a short article in the *Economist*, Bartleby describes teamwork as seen in a documentary on the Beatles. The following are some highlights from the column:

✳ "The Beatles documentary is a rare chance to watch a truly world-class team at work . . . Psychological makeup matters to how teams come together . . . Performance of groups is not correlated with their members' average intelligence but with characteristics such as sensitivity and how good teams are at giving everyone time to speak . . . and the ability to look here, there and everywhere for inspiration . . . and by the habit of keeping staleness at bay by taking risks, by learning from others and by innovating." Bartleby goes on to write, "Managers who think that building esprit de corps requires a separate activity from work—here comes the fun-time—are missing the point. The highest-performing TEAMs derive the greatest satisfaction not from each other, but from their work together" (119).

✳ As we have also seen, individuals supported in functioning as a team tend to have a more significant emotional investment and develop increasing ownership. As Dan Ariely says in Predictably Irrational "The more work you put into something, the more ownership you begin to feel for it" [(120) p. 175].

✳ There is often confusion about the scope of a team versus the meetings that most organizations regularly have. Meetings have gotten a bad rap, and in some organizations, they are disallowed. One of the hospital CEOs I worked with thought they were a total waste of time and ate up scarce resources better spent on other activities. In general, meetings are overdone, and in the modern communication age, utilizing the in-person time of twenty or thirty staff just to hear information is not worth the investment.

✳ In an article from Bloomberg Businessweek, Arianne Cohen summarizes tools proscribed by Neuroscientist Bruce Perry to get the most out of employees' brains. "Meetings are the dumbest thing any organization ever created. They default to a certain block of time and bring in a bunch of people to do nothing, while other parts of the organization are pressuring those people to be productive" (121).

✻ Team <u>working</u> sessions often mistitled as meetings, are distinctly different. These sessions bring people together to work on very focused and specific issues, with the invited having a vested interest. *They are essential in devising and implementing action.* Most of these people meet as frequently as weekly to establish a plan and engage appropriate stakeholders. After the first few conferences, the timing may be spaced out significantly, and communication and updates can be handled through technology. Although action-oriented and directed at staff, these gatherings must have senior leadership presence occasionally. This offers tacit support, active resource management, and encouragement and praise. In addition, it does provide executive leadership the opportunity to help coordinate these groups with more extensive organizational and operational plans.

✻ A team meeting, if structured appropriately, is an opportunity for staff to feel emotionally involved in determining processes and actions that they ultimately will be responsible for. As a team leader, some of the more successful meetings were when I could "keep my mouth closed" and listen to my peers and subordinates. My tacit role as a sponsor was important. Needing to meet my agenda was vital, but neither was as important as the trust and respect for my team members that my silence portrayed. This was one of the more difficult mechanisms as a leader, necessary to support the team and the individuals on it.

✻ The concept of a team made up of recognized individuals is essential in medicine but exists in many other organizations. Whether it is the almost unbelievable performance of the Blue Angels, or the fundamental safety inherent in crew resource management, the team is vital. A significant piece of my time as an executive was spent developing teams. Upfront, I can genuinely say that, even in comparison to emergently cracking a chest in the emergency department and saving a trauma victim, my team experiences were the most gratifying. Teaching, listening, learning from staff and colleagues, mentoring, and encouraging while demanding and observing the growth and commitment of a diverse team was both humbling and extremely rewarding.

OWNERSHIP

In Willink and Babin's book, the former SEALs discuss taking ultimate responsibility and *accountability* for their actions. They call this *extreme ownership*. (122) This does not come solely from understanding their role but from the commitment to their team, their nation, and the cause. They demonstrate this in a harrowing narrative of their wartime life and death experiences during the war in Iraq. Years of military experience, functioning as a team under the most adverse circumstances, and taking responsibility for the lives of their subordinates and teammates seem to be valuable ingredients for ownership.

Recognizing the need for ownership is more challenging to reproduce in the hospital setting. The elements of uncertainty and complexity in the acute care setting compared to the SEAL experience in Ramadi, Iraq, a violent insurgent-held city, seem a stretch. However, the message of the need for ownership and the barriers to achieving it highlights its importance in both settings.

Suppose the SEALs represent the ultimate team sport since their lives are dependent on each other. In that case, the acute hospital setting and its dependence on Team also have lives dependent on it, in the latter case, the lives of our patients.

Training and circumstances have embedded ownership into Unit Three's Task Force Bruiser members, not only in their dedicated leadership but also in every team member. Not only was their training focused on Ownership, but it was primarily cultivated over obvious interdependence, communication, and familiarity. Despite the heinous circumstances, decisions were made at all levels on the basis of trust in the system and each other.

In today's acute care setting, there has been a significant distinction between the described ownership in the SEALs ranks and what is visible in today's hospital environment. Patients often do not know who their care providers are. Inpatient hospitalists change frequently, nursing staff rotates based on three-day/week twelve-hour schedules, and there is increasing reliance on "tools" to take care of patients. Responsibility for care is scattered over many different individuals and specialties. It is not unusual for many members of the care team to change daily, in addition to the rotation of members on the day and night shifts. Additionally, the preponderance of sub-specialist involvement introduces another variable in the care pyramid.

As the intimacy of care and the physical interaction with our patients is further diluted by the time and focus on computer-based charts, diagnostic tests, compliance checklists, and the endless demand for increased documentation, it is rational to think that our ownership is also undermined. This ownership significantly comes usually from our direct involvement with patients, from conversations, sharing, starting IVs, giving medication to control pain to help with the first steps after surgery, and even from presenting bad news.

✱   Ariely in Predictably Irrational [(123) p. 169-178] discusses an "endowment effect that comes from owning something…. The more work you put into something, the more ownership you begin to feel for it." This ownership "increases the value or importance in the owners' eyes" and enhances their connection and focus on their immediate issues.

In some ways, this allows staff members to feel that their patient is akin to a family member, their "grandmother," and enhances the caring and attention to all the details of care.

When referring to a patient, it is always comforting to hear a nurse refer to "my patient in Room 12" rather than "the patient in Room 12." This slight difference suggests a different psychological connection. This starts a cascade that, as discussed, can have a powerful impact on error reduction and compliance with processes and tasks. This connection can also positively impact some social and personal biases that otherwise might undermine positive outcomes. A stranger is never a stranger in this type of environment.

On a more global scale, if we can facilitate making the copious amounts of data currently available to the same caregivers, and instead of merely being of interest, it starts to have a midbrain connection, our capabilities of positive change dramatically improve. Being aware of data is essential. Taking ownership of data and the **WHY** is the key to quality and safety at the micro-level.

In medical school, one was required to read, digest, and memorize thousands of details about anatomy, physiology, pharmacology, biochemistry, histology, and other arcane subjects. We all spent hundreds of hours pounding the books with variable success. Once we started hands-on clinical rotations and touched patients, the information became immediately personal and became part of an indelible learning base. The direct relationship with a patient allowed for the cascade of ownership, emotional midbrain connection, and subsequent intensity of learning.

A methodology that has met with some success currently is the establishment of *safety coaches*. The exact details of these positions may vary from facility to facility. Although their primary job is primary nursing care, they all capture these common themes.

- Advanced knowledge of safety and quality demands

- Understanding of the local needs and mores of their area

- On-the-ward/floor presence under normal working conditions

- Excellent communication skills

These coaches, taken from the active ranks of the clinical staff, are well accepted by their peers, and they model their ownership of individual safety and quality processes. They are the "local champion." Their activities often extend beyond safety and cross into quality areas.

One of the award-winning hospitals I associated with is just the right size. It is approximately a hundred beds in a community with less than average transiency. Serving as a regional hospital, it does have its share of drug/alcohol problems, homelessness, and psychiatric patients, but it is unique in its family feel. The staff is often put into a position to take care of family, neighbors, and friends. It is not unusual to be called out at the market or on the street by people you have cared for. This is the exact environment that amplifies endowment and ownership. What may not have been planned has become the standard, and with it being a hospital, we are all comfortable taking care of "Grandma."

When my kids were still small, we walked downtown, and my name was shouted across the busy main street. The voice was somewhat high-pitched and hysterical, and my kids looked alarmed. Finally, locating the vocalization source, my kids were stunned because it was a slightly disheveled individual showing outward signs and symptoms of chronic alcohol abuse. I walked across the street and returned the "knuckle handshake" offered to me and, after a few brief words, returned to my family time. "Who was that, Dad?" they wanted to know. I explained it was a patient I had taken care of several times in the emergency department and had tried to help.

Several years later, and after multiple visits to the hospital, the patient was admitted with a complex disease process that was ultimately fatal. I did not know he was in-house until members of the nursing staff called me and told me of his imminent demise. "We knew you would like to see him during this time, and he would like to see you."

He was not a member of my own family, but he was a member of the hospital and community family in a larger sense. These are the same nurses who refer to patients as "my patient." These are the same staff members who feel the ownership and accountability for each patient's care. This is the same staff that, when the quality and safety data is presented, including what they do every day, is not afraid to engage and try whatever it takes to make an impact. It is not incentive-based, nor even praise based. It is the intimacy of the staff with the patients, with each other, and with the community that drives them.

This particular hospital is an organic part of the community. The hospital board is made up of all types of community members that represent the geopolitics of the area. Although a not-for-profit hospital, the hospital itself significantly supports the one free clinic in the area. It donates yearly and contributes in-kind services, such as radiology, pathology studies, and even subspeciality operative services. I have been fortunate enough to be a founding member of this clinic's board. I have seen firsthand how the homeless and the undocumented receive no-questions-asked health, dental, and eye care.

Hector Alfonzo was a fifty-year-old man who was losing his eyesight to glaucoma. He had lived and worked in the United States for over twenty years. His three children had all been born locally, but he remained undocumented and unable to obtain medical benefits. He was evaluated and diagnosed at the free clinic, and an arrangement was made for a local ophthalmologist to evaluate him in his office. He needed emergent surgery to prevent blindness, and the hospital and the anesthesiology group agreed, after a bit of discussion, to donate their resources and their time. Hector's story has a happy ending, as he returned to work and was able to support his children long enough for them to graduate from high school.

It certainly is the size of the hospital and the geography of where it is located that encourages this level of intimacy. Still, it is also the culture and leadership at all levels that promulgate it. It is a recognition that must be imposed upon new employees and new "grad" nurses that have just completed nursing school. Remarkably, the hospital that did Hector's surgery has so many applicants for nursing jobs, since new nurses these days can almost go anywhere, they want. During interviews, so many candidates describe a family feeling that makes them want to work at this facility. It is not just warm and fuzzy. It promotes an atmosphere of ownership of the patients and accountability and commitment to each other, which ultimately is significantly responsible for award-winning care.

Ownership can have its dark side and must be kept in perspective not only in the patient care arena but also in the executive and leadership ranks. We discussed this in finance, where the feeling of ownership can influence investment decisions. Probably the best example of the potential negative influence of ownership comes from the movie *Bridge on the River Kwai*, based on the novel by Pierre Boulle. Alec Guinness, playing the British commander of a Japanese prison camp in WWII, is forced to lead his men in the arduous task of building a critical bridge to facilitate Japanese trains carrying essential supplies. His emotional sense of "ownership" of the bridge, based on a series of incredible hardships faced by him and his men, becomes so intense that he almost foils an allied attempt to destroy it. He finally realizes his error and dies in the process.

UNBALANCED

The value of the role of humans in the equation of medical care delivery is underestimated as we realize significant gains from new technologies. Even when the human element is mandatory, it is thought best to make it compliant with lists, rules, regulations, and standardized processes in direct patient care. It has been articulated that deviation from such is the cause of Human Error and is responsible for the multiple layers of mistakes and failures seen in our field.

As we have reviewed the recommendations of experts in the field, much of the articulated advances in health care are attributed to the scientific engineering of the daily processes. However, there can be little argument here that the role of humans in medicine demands a balance that recognizes that variability, uncertainty, complexity, urgency, and the unknown are intrinsic to our field. These elements require the involvement of all levels of staff in leadership, team, crew resource management, and decision-making, all toward patient care and the maintenance of active culture.

The balance of both sides of the equation allows for highly responsive care at the bedside and transformational thinking at the executive management level.

The themes discussed by A, E, I, O, and U have tremendous overlap and are difficult to separate in terms of methodology. The following table summarizes some of the key elements that describe the "state of the state." They are placeholders for considering how to restore balance in medicine as we bump along moving forward.

In each of the five areas within the table, the middle column reflects where we need to be and some of the elements, previously articulated, of how we can get there. The columns below utilize a few terms to suggest a culture that balances the current forces afield that can lead to organizational excellence.

AWARENESS	Teams	WHY, not WHAT
	Meetings	Projections
	Rounds	Perfection cannot be the goal
	Data selection & prioritization	Active culture
	Champions & Coaches	
ENGAGEMENT	Leadership	Ownership
	Communications	Accountability
	Enhance direct contact with patients	Midbrain connection
	& staff	Intimacy
	Don't settle for comput-	Continuity
	er-based communication	Loyalty
	Reduce substitutions	
INDIVIDUAL	Personalized data	Stress 4 success
	Understand bias	Leadership
	Rewards, support, and recognition	Attachment
	Decision vortex	Personal growth
		Emotional intelligence
OWNERSHIP	Trust	Fully integrated outpatient system (clin-
	Whole person care	ics, post-acute, surgery centers)
	Care coordination across	
	the continuum	
(UN) BALANCED	Focus on goals, not tools	Embrace technology without abandoning
	AI vs Connection	the Hippocratic Oath
	Local vs System decisions	Quadruple aim
	One size does not fit all	

Writing about **WHAT2WHY** and all of the five **Ws** was an opportunity to organize my thinking about what exactly is the bottom line, where are we at in medicine, where are we going, and are there lessons from other industries that could help us move forward.

Additionally, are their lessons from our own trials and tribulations that provide insight that is then transferable to other endeavors outside of taking care of patients?

We are blessed with more *knowledge* about what we do than ever before. Some of us believe that we are under a microscope that will show every flaw, but the reality is the type of business we are in must self-examine ourselves honestly and openly. The following is the entire poem, a piece of which was seen in the table of contents, from T. S. Eliot, "The Rock," 1934:

> All our knowledge brings us near to our ignorance,
>
> All our ignorance brings us nearer to death,
>
> Nearness to death, no nearer to God.
>
> Where is the Life we have lost in living?
>
> Where is the wisdom we have lost in knowledge?
>
> Where is the knowledge we have lost in information?
>
> The cycles of Heaven in twenty centuries
>
> Bring us farther from God and nearer to the Dust.

Without getting too philosophical, Eliot underscores how focusing on information, data, percentages, or grades may have a deleterious effect. Information is but a waypoint in our quest. Engaging foremost in the process of analytics and in-depth clinical review can assist in information becoming knowledge. This knowledge then can become the jumping-off point for action. Yet it is the ownership of this knowledge that allows humans to broadly develop the skills and the drive to integrate wisdom into action.

The Oxford Dictionary defines "wisdom" as:
- "The quality of having experience, knowledge and good judgment"

- "The soundness of an action or decision concerning the application of experience, knowledge and good judgment"

✴ The final **W** is what to do about it and the action necessary to make it happen, where intuition, experience, and sound judgment are the key elements. This wisdom differentiates us from total dependence on artificial intelligence. This wisdom allows us to honestly care for our patients and each other.

✴ The bottom line should not be our profit and loss statement, bond rating, EBITDA (Earnings Before Interest, Taxes, Depreciation and Amortization), or even publicly reported grades. Wisdom differentiates the human elements from the tools, no matter how far advanced, and is the fundamental element of quality and safety in medicine.

I hope I have been able to express the principal factors that have caused an unbalance in my field. I have done this without animus and not without an appreciation of the monumental progress that many of the same elements have brought in patient care. I fully understand that I live in a *meta-universe* and that many of the applications that I find unnerving are reflections of what is going on in the world around us. I also understand that the many new individuals entering my field have a very different telescope. Their experience and even their education have prepared them for a very different medical environment.

I do not thirst for the old days when, for example, 80+ percent of pediatric patients with leukemia died (The current rate is 20 percent or less.). I do not yearn for the isolationism of American medicine, the vast discrepancies of care between countries and even socio-economic groups, some of which have become more of a focus during the current pandemic.

✔ I admit to wanting to hold on to some values that continue to exemplify that we are still *humans taking care of humans*. As such, we are tempered by our own histories and experiences and the culture and environment where we find ourselves. Even Dr. Leonard McCoy from *Star Trek* and his *tricorder* in the last part of the twenty-second century was still characterized by his intimate personal/psychological involvement with his patients and crew. His ability to connect with his crewmates and the patients that came under his care made him uniquely qualified, not the blinking, noisy diagnostic tool in his hand.

✶ We have stepped away from the bedside and no longer rely upon or even utilize a hands-on physical exam. We rather rely on our high-end diagnostics and accept a transient relationship with most of our patients. We are satisfied with a communication system that discourages in-person discussion with our colleagues, staff, and patients. Many of the sophisticated diagnostic tests we order are so specialized that we do not even attempt our own interpretation but rely on distal readings by a specialist entered into the computer-based medical record. Continuity of care is as rare as hen's teeth, although we have made efforts, but committed limited resources, to fill in those gaps.

✶ Being under the microscope has spawned an entire data science industry, giving us thousands of data points about our compliance with standardized processes but often only code- and documentation-based outcome data. Quality and safety scientists have promulgated distinct but overlapping methodologies that frequently try to eliminate human judgment and decision-making from the equation. Their basic approach is to limit the opportunities for human error. Perhaps a more reasonable system is to balance this scientific approach with an understanding of the need for intimacy and human behavior. The ability to empathize enhances our ability to communicate with patients and helps us *own* the very focused care we provide. This ownership helps us not make mistakes or failures in following best practices because, after all, it is "Grandma."

✶ The team cannot exist if its only purpose is to follow the rules. The investment of time, energy, and resources required to be an owner make our efforts real. We have spent multiple years trying to deliver validated, prioritized, and analyzed *data* to the folks in the trenches. Sitting in a meeting, or receiving computer-based printouts, may pique interest. However, suppose there is a process to integrate the doers in the active awareness, understanding, and data analysis of their own and teams' performance. In that case, you can imagine the different intensities of response. The closer we can provide data and insight to the bedside in a real-time frame, the more impact we can expect— the more engaged the team, the more creativity, problem-solving, and *action* we can expect.

What humans bring to the table is admittedly sometimes problematic. Bias, mainly unrecognized bias, may cloud judgment. The balance in decision-making between data and algorithm and emotional intelligence and intuition can significantly impact a patient's life. The inherent humanness of a caregiver can be variously problematic in critical decisions, especially those made rapidly, without complete information and analysis, in the chaos and uncertainty of the acute care hospital. Yet within the "guardrails" of engineered processes and redundancy, these human elements can and should be recognized for their effectiveness. A proper understanding of ourselves, who we are and how we got here, putting in perspective our experience and pattern recognition that develops intuition, can be the essential element of organizational excellence.

Extracting human elements from the mix seems to be a trend in planning and our essential human nature. The dependence on technology and its demands and needs makes our human interactions and skills less of a priority. We are rewarded more for compliance than for commitment. Incentives are based more on mathematics than on skills and overall care delivery. And the incentives are almost always financial, based on formulas rather than an accurate recognition of our abilities and performance.

Dr. Millson was an older internist at an immense tertiary care teaching hospital in a major West Coast city. Like many of the internists of his day, he liked to follow his own patients, even when they were hospitalized. He continued to read and study, go to conferences, and stay abreast with current trends and technology changing the field. No surprise, his patients loved him, many of whom had been with him for a lifetime.

One late night, or more precisely around 3:00 a.m., when working in the ED, one of his patients came in with an acute myocardial infarction. Dr. Millson appeared after the patient was stabilized in the ED and the emergency heart catheterization team mobilized. By this point, the cardiology fellow and several residents were busy preparing for the patient's emergency heart catheterization. Still, Millson went to the patient's bedside, sat down, reached out for the patient's forearm, not being used to starting IVs, and quietly talked to him amid the urgent activity around him.

Within fifteen minutes, the patient was wheeled off to the catheterization lab, and Dr. Millson came to the doctor's station in the middle of the main treatment area of the ED and sat down. "First, I want to thank you," he said. "The patient wanted you to know that he appreciated your timely care and concern." His comment touched me and I said, "You and I have shared many patients over the last few years. Didn't you trust that I would take good care of him?" "Of course, I did," he said," but he has been *my patient* for some time, and I wanted to be here for him." We talked about why he was in the ED at 3:00 a.m., which we both laughed about, and then he told me he was retiring.

I told him I was sad to see him go, but that I understood, that because of his age and health, it was probably the best decision, but that I would personally miss him and that the most significant loss, apart from his patients, would be for the resident house staff. "You are really one of the few role models that remain in our rapidly changing medical world," I said. "You care about your patients, and they feel it. Whether in your office, the ED, rehab, or back home, you own them. The continuity you provide is perhaps more essential than you even realize. I just want to thank you for all you have done for your patients, the community, this hospital, your peers, and our next generation of caregivers."

⚕ The continuity of care that was a stable in Dr. Millson's practice has become much more complex to provide for our patients. Not impossible, but it now requires a well-resourced, coordinated team functioning cooperatively within all the varied elements of a care system. Whole patient care may be a new buzzword in our lexicon, but as our medical system changes, the quest for continuity must be its *keystone*.

⚕⚕ A balance between the phenomenal advances in technology and that medicine is still about *humans taking care of humans* is essential for our future. This message must be delivered and modeled at every opportunity for all new people matriculating into our field. Even more important is the reminder of this assertion to the current care providers. Doctors, nurses, and others are being swept into a situation where most of their time, energy, and focus is channeled into a *video-game mentality*. The new reality appears on their screen, and life and death only contribute to the nominal score of winning or losing.

The Hippocratic Oath has long been seen as the rock bed of professional ethics and taught by multiple generations of "healers." The original version of the Oath has been updated since its original Greek version, most recently in the 1960s. When surveyed in 2000, of the US medical schools, 122 still used the Hippocratic Oath or a modernized version.

One of the key components of the Hippocratic Oath:

- "I will remember that there is an art to medicine as well as science, and that warmth, sympathy and understanding may outweigh the surgeon's knife or the chemist's drug."

As caregivers, our DNA goes back to the original cave drama described in the very initial part of this book. Medical schools have worked diligently to continue to impart the feeling of ownership, responsibility, and accountability to our patients. Nevertheless, we now increasingly refer to "the patient" rather than "my patient," and technology has firmly reinforced the chiasm. The oath above becomes more and more outdated by the predominant focus on diagnostic and therapeutic tools and our overwhelming relationship with the electronic medical record.

I have discussed many issues critical to our future in the previous pages. I freely admit my bias about health care, particularly the hospital experience. The considerations mentioned above are not directed only at institutional change or angst about the current corporate practice of medicine, although fine-tuning patient care, which I believe is a *local responsibility*, is more and more challenging to accomplish in isolation.

Without the ability to practice in multiple states, negotiate financial remuneration with the government and health insurance payors, and have a meaningful discussion with multiple different unions, the job of a health care system is doomed for failure. In a not-for-profit situation, where I have spent the majority of my history, it is also essential to go to national financial resources for bonds that allow for the continuous need for expanding resources and investment in new and costly state-of-the-art technology.

Despite this corporate rationale, it is often more difficult to appreciate how the concept of scale in a vast national health system benefits the local hospitals. Standardization, with little regard to local community needs, both from the medical and social points of view, often stimulates conflicts of interest amongst the prevailing stakeholders. It is difficult to embrace the idea that large health care systems have moved the goal of excellent patient care behind success, or at least stability, efficiency, compliance, and even growth.

Large national health care systems have a serious choice of approaches to improving health care in their national market. They can focus on the lessons of excellence in their best-performing markets and resource the poorest performers to drive for improvement. This approach can facilitate a shift of the average system-wide performance reflected in their bell-shaped curve to the right.

The other approach utilized by some national health systems is to adopt aims primarily to improve the average system performance by standardization for all hospitals toward the middle of the bell-shaped curve. Admittedly, this focuses improvement on those facilities on the left of the curve, moving them statistically toward the center, but also then moves the outstanding performers to the middle of the curve.

The other consideration about future health care puts the responsibility firmly on us humans. Increasingly social determinants of health are more significant than our excellent diagnostic and therapeutic modalities in improving the health care ills of our society. Our ability to respond to our time's overarching issues, such as homelessness, drug/alcohol abuse, severely limited psychiatric resources, abuse, neglect, and exploitation, challenge our limited medical resources.

The reluctance of our society to deal with end-of-life issues is disrespectful to both the living and the dying. A good percentage of our health care dollars is committed to patients in the last six or even three months of their lives.

Patients and their families demand unnecessary and ineffective treatments. *Palliative care* is now available at most hospitals and in post-acute situations and clinics and even in some private physician offices. This is not simply to offer and discuss hospice care, which it can do, but to introduce the concept of *goals of care*. This conversation is not necessarily only about end-of-life issues but about the patient's illness, the potential therapies, and making informed decisions about care options and what they mean to the patient and the family. Unfortunately, a good portion of patients that ultimately elect hospice care does so only in their last week of life. Hospice agencies have so much more to offer to patients and their families.

Many patient families will go so far as to hide serious or terminal news from their loved ones.

"Doctor, are you sure there are no other treatments available?" the patient's daughter asked. "Should we take her to the university medical center again?"

"We have her on the university experimental protocol, and unfortunately, it does not appear to be working. The pain from her metastasis is increasing," the cancer specialist replied.

"I want everything done to fight the cancer," the daughter said tearfully.

"I want the palliative care nurse to see Mom," said the doctor. "She can help with pain control and support Mom in dealing with her condition," the doctor replied.

"No, absolutely not. We are not putting her in hospice until the last minute, or ever," the daughter replies in tears.

Most patients and their families don't understand the difference between hospice and palliative care. The latter is an opportunity to discuss goals of care much before the terminal phase of an illness. It empowers patients in dealing with inevitable events and is very supportive physiologically and psychologically. Many patients refuse to see palliative care personnel to avoid the discussion of DNR (Do Not Resuscitate) or POLST (Physician Orders for Life-Sustaining Treatment) that better proscribe medical care in end-of-life events). Sometimes even shared erroneously by doctors, this decision is a tremendous disservice to patients.

Hospice care is perhaps the best example of humans taking care of humans. The love and respect they provide patients and their expertise in pain control is a significant benefit during the last months of life. Hospice helps reduce pain and suffering, both physically and emotionally. Cancer physicians seem to understand the role of palliative care and hospice fully. Some specialists, such as cardiologists and lung doctors, who have more and more advanced tools, seem to struggle with accepting the positive impact of ✓ palliative care programs.ospice Palliative and hospice care does not mean *no treatment*, which is a popular misconception that must be put to rest.

An even more important consideration is the health care decisions made by humans, significantly outside the control of providers and hospitals. These ✗ decisions are made owing to habit, ignorance, and disregard. Cigarette smoking is one example. It was understandable at some level that smoking was promulgated by actors and the movies in the 1940s and 1950s. It was cool to smoke. In some situations, it was even recommended by physicians. There were several generations of people who ended their lives very uncomfortably from the effects of smoking. They did not know the damage and predisposition to cancer that smoking tobacco produced until they were habituated. Fast forward to current times, when the information about smoking and chronic lung disease and the predisposition for cancer and heart disease are well known. The fastest segment of growth of smoking in our population is adolescents.

Unfortunately, *vaccination* is another issue that has become highly polarized owing to regional, social, and political influence that has undoubtedly complicated the global response to Covid-19 and other contagious illnesses. The news media publishes a significant difference in vaccination and death rates when blue and red states are compared. Politics has undoubtedly impacted me even in my little corner of the world. It seems that only when illness strikes and even kill close to home are the terrible consequences seen daily in hospitals to both staff and patients recognized on a "gut level." Even something as simple as measles vaccination has met serious resistance in pockets of our country.

⚹ Some of the issues faced in today's health care are complicated by state-by-state and federal legislation that is variable and often politically driven that complicating patients' care. All but a few states allow hospitals actually to employ physicians. A few, like California, prevent physicians from being employed by hospitals because of the fear that physicians under the control of hospitals would admit patients unnecessarily. Most facilities get around this legislation by contracting with doctors to provide services, but this adds to the complexity financially and the potential adherence and enforcement of hospital rules and regulations.

⚺ Another complication is that some well-meaning state legislative actions interfere with best practice performance. An example is the advanced HIPAA or privacy regulations impacting drug and alcohol-addicted patients. It makes sense that patients seeking addiction care in rehabilitation facilities are very protected regarding their privacy. It is problematic that these patients admitted to acute care hospitals for medical issues must keep information about their addiction and the advice of addiction specialists in a separate and view-limited record available to only a few people. As you can imagine, having two medical records for a single patient is a potential safety issue, and limiting an addiction specialist's advice to a separate document, not open to the physicians taking primary care of the patient, is very problematic.

Despite many conversations and efforts to simplify these issues, the circumstances still exist, as legal thinking sometimes takes precedence over patients' most appropriate and safe care.

The medical community, hospitals, care providers, and outpatient facilities are one leg of a *three-legged stool* that makes up medical care today. The second leg is the government (state and federal) and private payors that make the rules and determine compensation for care. The third leg is us, humans.

✓ We need to do a better job moving forward in coordination, collaboration, and cooperation, or one or all of the legs will cave with very predictable results.

The social determinants of disease, which I described earlier, are emerging as perhaps the most significant impediment to community health care. The issues complicating a response to the homeless crisis are making coordinated action nearly impossible. Sponsored mobile showers, free clinics, tiny homes, expanded rescue shelters, and many other significant ideas have all helped. However, as long as NIMBY (not in my backyard) is a community theme and all the elements it represents, a coordinated approach is nearly impossible. The idea that homelessness has so many reasons should not invalidate a system that prioritizes a response to each element, ideally in collaboration.

I have now "barked" at everyone for not taking responsibility for ourselves and the planet. I am hopeful that the influence can, in some way, balance all the negative issues articulated about corporate medicine that its size may offer. Influence on drug companies, legislatures, insurance behemoths, and government agencies such as CMS can lead to a more inclusive positive collaboration. This would represent a tremendous step forward and might even have significant financial and operational benefits for everyone involved.

✓ Finally, striving to incorporate our human aspects, such as ownership of our patients, never losing that focus, despite the seduction and promise of technology, leaves me a little more hopeful for future healthcare generations.

Hopefully, projecting our future in medicine will encompass the themes from the previous discussions in this book. I hope it will showcase a medical culture of humans taking care of humans, endowed with empathy, accountability, and ownership. I want to think that understanding the essentials of a team will be an essential aspect of how we move forward, reflecting that quality and safety are not merely grades or scores, but that they help us understand the opportunities we have to make a real difference in the care of our patients.

I have presented some tools that have worked for my teams and me to enable us to make serious progress and improvements. Underscore, please, the great pleasure and satisfaction I have had from empowering individuals, watching them grow and becoming leaders in their own right. I hope I have presented some insights into bias, confirmational bias, and how it complicates our decisions every day in our complex and rapidly changing and uncertain world.

Many of the themes and structures I have discussed are the health care world insights. Still, I believe they have an application to many other industries, particularly those who realize that *people are their most important resource*. Unfortunately, I have had to reflect on how trends, although important, can undermine essential aspects of what I hold dear.

There is a forgone conclusion that all industries at some level will embrace working from home. The projections are for the prevalence of a hybridized model. Rebecca Penty in Bloomberg Businessweek has stated, "Allowing working from home not only increases productivity slightly but also markedly improves employee retention rates, giving organizations all the motivation, they need to let employees log on" (124). It would be reasonable to consider that the acute care hospital defies this scheme regarding patient care. However, remote connections with patients made a significant impact on our clinic systems, particularly during the worst times of the pandemic. It taught a generation of patients with mobility issues the ease and comfort of telehealth.

Offsite monitoring is increasingly available. In smaller hospitals trying to maintain 24/7 coverage in their intensive care units, contracted off-site monitoring and physician coverage has been used to fill gaps. Home monitoring of chronically ill patients is also increasingly available, facilitated by technological progress. The future of these new processes accelerated in part by the pandemic will continue to impact patients, even as the Covid pandemic retreats.

VIII.
PROJECTION
AND REFLECTION

The balance between AI, impressive technological advances, the impact of the centralized corporate approach to medicine, and that of humans taking care of humans is severely threatened.

Closing my eyes and projecting medicine in the not-too-distant future is quite worrisome.

Jonathan Jones, a forty-five-year-old man in the future, plagued with a bothersome cough, used his cell phone to access his health care provider. Previously he would have been asked to insert his identifying information and a PIN uniquely issued to him. He is requested on this occasion to stare with one eye into his phone's camera lens. There is a red light for him to focus on. An iris scan confirms his identity and automatically his medical record is consulted.

After only a few brief seconds, a banner of the Forrest Health Care System (there is none such) appears on the phone and welcomes him personally by his name. Shortly after that, an *avatar* appears, depicting an attractive middle-aged woman.

> "Welcome, Jonathan Jones," she says and smiles warmly. "I am your doctor's virtual medical assistant immediately available to you because Forrest Health cares about you."

After a few seconds of speechlessness, Jones replies, "I am supposed to check in with my doctor about my persistent cough."

"That is correct, Mr. Jones," the avatar replies. "I have the test results that I will share with you, but can you first hold your handheld device, ensuring that both thumbs are touching the screen, please?"

Jonathan fumbles a little but feels a very low, not unpleasant, electrical current and holds his thumbs in place as directed.

"I now have your EKG and, in a few seconds, will have your blood test results as well, derived from your thumbs touching your phone," the avatar states.

"That's amazing," Jonathan says, "all from that little electrical activity from the phone. No waiting, no getting blood drawn, or waiting long periods for someone available to do my EKG."

"That's correct," the avatar responds with a smile, "all because Forrest Health cares.

"She then says, "We have reviewed your results from the mobile radiology van that we sent to your house, and I will give you those results after you answer a few simple questions for the medical record, which is being documented as we speak. How do you feel, on a scale of 1 to 10, with ten being the best?" the avatar says. "Are your symptoms the same or increasing, on a scale of 1 to 10? Is your cough productive? 1 for yes, 2 for no."

The avatar smiles and makes direct eye contact with the patient. "Your X-ray shows a 73 percent probability that your cough is coming from simple pneumonia but will be reviewed by a specialist to rule out other possibilities."

"Should I be worried about pneumonia or the 'other possibilities"? Jonathan asks.

"We have prescribed an antibiotic, which your record shows you have no allergies to, and this will be delivered directly to your address by a drone within the next three hours. Please press 1 to confirm that you have no allergies to this medication, or press 2 if there have been issues in the past usage. Your screening blood evaluation today shows mildly elevated blood sugar. Please move the camera on your phone very close to your eye and do not blink in the bright light you will see," the avatar instructs.

After a few seconds, the avatar said, "We have looked at your retina and do not see any evidence of diabetes at this time, but it is one of the things we will follow up on. I will call you within the next seventy-two hours to see how you are doing," the avatar says pleasantly, "because Forrest Health cares. Please call me if your symptoms worsen or you have trouble taking the medication. Also, please call in in the next thirty days, and we will check your blood sugar and other tests to rule out diabetes."

Though somewhat flabbergasted by the entire phone process, Jonathan thanks the avatar, unsure if that was the appropriate reaction.

She says, "Your medical records are available simply by utilizing your iris scan. Goodbye."

Some of the problematic issues I have commented upon that have developed in my field over the last decades are answered by this "brave new world" of technology. Continuity issues have been addressed with the addition of telehealth and the enhanced capabilities of the Internet.

Utilizing iris scans and retinal scans for identification and diagnosis are already available at some airports and ophthalmology offices. It is not much of a jump to see their applications available on a cell phone, as it was with Jonathan.

Jonathan's commitment to his care has been reinforced by reducing the barriers and steps usually present when accessing care. His conversation with the avatar, his diagnostics, and even his medications require minimal complex physical action on his part. Forrest Health saves massive dollars in physician/provider time and improves access for more complicated, sicker patients.

Does Jonathan feel cared for, despite the repetition by the avatar of Forrest Health's goals? Is the avatar capable of showing empathy or understanding the patient's position? Is it important? Where is the "wisdom" from a provider that calls Jonathan "my patient"?

In previous pages, I commented on the seductiveness of advancing technologies. When I discussed this with one of my colleagues, a well-known recently retired cardio-vascular surgeon, "That train has already left the station" was his comment.

Heath, C. &Heath, D, in their book Switch(125) describe how to change things when change is hard.

Many of the forces in medicine that we are faced with today add to the complexity and uncertainty of far-reaching decisions. I have tried in the book to embrace change without eliminating those attributes that make taking care of patients unique. Our uncertainties cannot allow us to stagnate since our patients depend on us, "Until you can ladder your way down from a change idea to a specific behavior, you're not ready to lead a switch. To create movement, you have got to be specific and concrete." (126) We have the tools to do this, but should never lose sight of our ultimate goal, and the why we are doing what we are doing. Sometimes specific tools lead to very narrow solutions and the challenge is to balance our approach and continually focus on the fact "that one size does not fit all".

Another trap that larger health care systems fall into is centralism of thought. In his article After Babel in the Atlantic Monthly Jonathan Haidt says, "The most pervasive obstacle to good thinking is confirmation bias, which refers to the human tendency to search only for evidence that confirms our preferred beliefs." (127) As discussed earlier in the book this can disrupt every type of situation from the bedside to the national boardroom. Haidt goes on to further say," The most reliable cure for confirmation bias is interacting who don't share your beliefs. They confront you with counterevidence and counterarguments." (128)

Bolman and Deal in their book Reframing Organizations (129) state "There is no one best way to organize. The right structure depends on the prevailing circumstances and considers an organization's goals, strategies, technology, people and environment." Reaching the ultimate goal requires an understanding and balance of all these factors.

Medicine will continue to change even in the immediate future. Great discoveries push us forward. Gene sequencing and enhanced computer capabilities portend the possibility of not only projecting potential illness but manipulating it. Today we see our behemoth national corporations such as Amazon and Walmart developing new types of patient access, and looking to design entirely unique care experiences.

I hope that we recognize that care is more than a process as we move forward. We can advance mightily with the help of technology without losing the humanness and balance in what we do. I hope that the future generation of caregivers will have the opportunity to derive the humbling satisfaction from what we do, which I have been privileged to experience.

REFERENCES

(1) Haggard, Howard, <u>The Doctor in History</u>, Dorset Press, 1989. page 9

(2) Haggard, Howard, <u>The Doctor in History</u>, Dorset Press, 1989. page 65

(3) Kahneman, Daniel, <u>Thinking Fast and Slow</u>, Farrar, Straus and Giroux, 2011.

(4) Garvey-Berger J., <u>Changing on the Job</u>, Stanford University Press, 2012. Pg 120

(5) Garvey-Berger J., <u>Changing on the Job</u>, Stanford University Press, 2012. Pg 120

(6) Sommers, Sam, <u>Situations Matter</u>, Riverhead Books, 2011. pg. 17

(7) Schein, Edgar H., <u>Organizational Culture and Leadership</u>, John Wiley & Sons, Inc., 2017.

(8) Platts-Mills, T. et al., <u>Tolerance of Uncertainty and the Practice of Emergency Medicine</u>, Annals of Emergency Medicine, Volume 75, No. 6 June 2020, p715-720.

(9) Clapper, C., Merlino, J., Stockmeier, <u>Zero Harm</u>, McGraw Hill, 2019.

(10) Clapper, C., Merlino, J., Stockmeier, <u>Zero Harm</u>, McGraw Hill, 2019, p 243

(11) Clapper, C., Merlino, J., Stockmeier, <u>Zero Harm</u>, McGraw Hill, 2019.

(12) Gawande, Atul, <u>Being Mortal</u>, Metropolitan Books, 2014., p 6

(13) Gawande, Atul, <u>Being Mortal</u>, Metropolitan Books, 2014., p 3

(14) Gawande, Atul, <u>Being Mortal</u>, Metropolitan Books, 2014., p 1

(15) Coget, J-F, Keller, E., <u>The Critical Decision Vortex</u>, Journal of Management Inquiry, 2010.

(16) Gladwell, Malcolm, <u>Blink, the Power of Thinking Without Thinking</u>, Little Brown & Company, Jan. 2005.

(17) Goleman, Daniel, <u>Emotional Intelligence</u>, Bantum Books, October 1995.

(18) Lewis, Michael, <u>The Undoing Project</u>, W. W. Norton, 2017, p 190.

(19) Kahneman, Daniel, <u>Thinking Fast and Slow</u>, Farrar, Straus and Giroux, 2011.

(20) Kahneman, Daniel, <u>Thinking Fast and Slow</u>, Farrar, Straus and Giroux, 2011, p 237

(21) Gladwell, Malcolm, <u>Blink, the Power of Thinking Without Thinking</u>, Little Brown & Company, Jan. 2005.

(22) Lewis, Michael, <u>The Undoing Project</u>, W. W. Norton, 2017. p 256.

(23) Lewis, Michael, <u>The Undoing Project</u>, W. W. Norton, 2017, p 261

(24) Lewis, Michael, <u>The Undoing Project</u>, W. W. Norton, 2017, p 261

(25) Gawande, Atul, <u>The Checklist Manifesto</u>, METROPOLITAN Books Henry Holt and Co., 2009, p 13.

(26) Gawande, Atul, <u>The Checklist Manifesto</u>, METROPOLITAN Books Henry Holt and Co., 2009, p 13

(27) Goleman, Daniel, <u>Working with Emotional Intelligence</u>, Bantam Books, 1998, p 135

(28) Goleman, Daniel, <u>Emotional Intelligence</u>, Bantum Books, October 1995.

(29) Goleman, Daniel, <u>Working with Emotional Intelligence</u>, Bantam Books, 1998, p 23.

(30) Goleman, Daniel, <u>Working with Emotional Intelligence</u>, Bantam Books, 1998, p 26.

(31) Baer, Tobias. Schnall, Simone, <u>Quantifying the Cost of Decision Fatigue: Suboptimal Risk   Decisions in Finance</u>, The Royal Society Open Science, Issue 5, May 2021.

(32) Goleman, Daniel, <u>Emotional Intelligence</u>, Bantum Books, October 1995, p 139

(33) Bungay, S., <u>The Art of Action</u>, Nicholas Brealey Publishing, 2011.

(34)

(35) Goleman, Daniel, <u>Working with Emotional Intelligence</u>, Bantam Books, 1998, p 139

(36) Schein, Edgar H., <u>Organizational Culture and Leadership</u>, John Wiley & Sons, Inc., 2017, p 4.

(37) Kenney, Charles, <u>Transforming Health Care</u>, CRC Press, 2011.

(38) Schein, Edgar H., <u>Organizational Culture and Leadership</u>, John Wiley & Sons, Inc., 2017.

(39) Sinek, S., <u>Start with Why</u>, Portfolio/Penguin, 2009, p 142

(40) Sinek, S., <u>Start with Why</u>, Portfolio/Penguin, 2009, p 6

(41) Kouzes, James & Posner, Barry, <u>The leadership Challenge</u>, Jossey-Bass, A Wiley Company, p 22

(42) Sinek, S., <u>Start with Why</u>, Portfolio/Penguin, 2009, p 22

(43) Sinek, S., <u>Start with Why</u>, Portfolio/Penguin, 2009, p 104

(44) Frisina, Michael E., <u>Influential leadership</u>, Health Administration Press, 2011, p 24.

(45) Frisina, Michael E., Influential leadership, Health Administration Press, 2011, p 27.

(46) Gladwell, Malcolm, Blink, the Power of Thinking Without Thinking, Little Brown & Company, Jan. 2005.

(47) Myers, David G., Exploring Social Psychology, McGraw Hill, 2009, p 71.

(48) Goleman, D, Boyatzis, R. & McKee, A., Primal Leadership, Harvard Business Review Press, 2013, p 38.

(49) Goleman, D, Boyatzis, R. & McKee, A., Primal Leadership, Harvard Business Review Press, 2013, p 28.

(50) Frisina, Michael E., Influential leadership, Health Administration Press, 2011, p 27.

(51) Penty, Rebecca & Begun, Bret, Goodbye Plan, Hello Scenarios, Bloomberg Businessweek, Feb. 14, 2022 p. 34-35.

(52) Penty, Rebecca & Begun, Bret, Goodbye Plan, Hello Scenarios, Bloomberg Businessweek, Feb. 14, 2022 p. 34-35.

(53) Deal, Terrence, Bolman, Lee G., Reframing Organizations, John Wiley & Sons, 2008. Pg 69

(54) Deal, Terrence, Bolman, Lee G., Reframing Organizations, John Wiley & Sons, 2008. Pg 41.

(55) Penty, Rebecca & Begun, Bret, Goodbye Plan, Hello Scenarios, Bloomberg Businessweek, Feb. 14, 2022 p. 34-35.

(56) Sinek, S., Start with Why, Portfolio/Penguin, 2009.

(57) Cuddy, A., Presence, Little Brown Spark, Hachette Book Group, 2015, p 76.

(58) Sinek, S., Start with Why, Portfolio/Penguin, 2009, p 55.

(59) Sinek, S., <u>Start with Why</u>, Portfolio/Penguin, 2009, p 56.

(60) Kahneman, Daniel., Sibony, Oliver, Sunstein, Casss R., <u>Noise</u>, Hachette Book Group, 2021.p.169

(61) Matta, Christy, <u>The Stress Response</u>, New Harbinger Publications, 2012.

(62) Loehr, James E., <u>Stress for Success</u>, Random House, 1997.

(63) Platts-Mills, T. et al., <u>Tolerance of Uncertainty and the Practice of Emergency Medicine</u>, Annals of Emergency Medicine, Volume 75, No. 6 June 2020, p715-720.

(64) Weick, Karl, Sutcliffe, Kathleen M., <u>Managing the Unexpected</u>, John Wiley & Sons, 2015.

(65) Chodren, Pema, <u>Comfortable with Uncertainty</u>, 108 Teachings, August 13, 2002.

(66) Haidt, Jonathen, <u>After Babel</u>, The Atlantic, May 2022. Pg 60.

(67) Gawande, Atul, <u>The Checklist Manifesto</u>, METROPOLITAN Books Henry Holt and Co., 2009, p 13.

(68) Chodren, Pema, <u>Comfortable with Uncertainty</u>, 108 Teachings, August 13, 2002, p 5.

(69) Gleick, James, <u>Chaos</u>, Penguin Books, 2008, p 279.

(70) Kahneman, Daniel, <u>Thinking Fast and Slow</u>, Farrar, Straus and Giroux, 2011.

(71) Lewis, Michael, <u>The Undoing Project</u>, W. W. Norton, 2017.

(72) Kahneman, Daniel., Sibony, Oliver, Sunstein, Casss R., <u>Noise</u>, Hachette Book Group, 2021.p.169

(73) Webb, Alex, <u>Big Tech's New Vision</u>, Bloomberg Businessweek,December 20, 2021, p.10-11

(74) Bodenheimer T, Sinsky C., <u>From Triple to Quadruple Aim</u>, Ann Fam Medicine 2014:12:573-76.

(75) Wears, R. L., Sutcliffe, K., <u>Still Not Safe</u>, Oxford University Press, 2020.

(76) Clapper, C., Merlino, J., Stockmeier, <u>Zero Harm,</u> McGraw Hill, 2019.

(77) Clapper, C., Merlino, J., Stockmeier, <u>Zero Harm,</u> McGraw Hill, 2019.

(78) Clapper, C., Merlino, J., Stockmeier, <u>Zero Harm,</u> McGraw Hill, 2019, p 103.

(79) Kahneman, Daniel, <u>Thinking Fast and Slow</u>, Farrar, Straus and Giroux, 2011, p 98.

(80) Reason, James, <u>Human Error</u>, Cambridge University Press, 1990.

(81) Reason, James, <u>Human Error</u>, Cambridge University Press, 1990.

(82) Reason, James, <u>Human Error</u>, Cambridge University Press, 1990.

(83) Clapper, C., Merlino, J., Stockmeier, <u>Zero Harm,</u> McGraw Hill, 2019.

(84) Reason, James, <u>Human Error</u>, Cambridge University Press, 1990.

(85) Wears, R. L., Sutcliffe, K., <u>Still Not Safe</u>, Oxford University Press, 2020.

(86) Lehrer, Jonah, <u>How We Decide</u>, Houghton Mifflin Harcourt Publishing Company, 2009.

(87) Lehrer, Jonah, <u>How We Decide</u>, Houghton Mifflin Harcourt Publishing Company, 2009, p 18.

(88) Penty, Rebecca & Begun, Bret<u>, Goodbye Plan, Hello Scenarios,</u> Bloomberg Businessweek, Feb. 14, 2022 p. 34-35.

(89) Wears, R. L., Sutcliffe, K., <u>Still Not Safe</u>, Oxford University Press, 2020, p 43.

(90) Wears, Robert & Sutcliffe, Kathleen M., <u>Still Not Safe</u>, Oxford University Press, 2020,p 42.

(91) Wears, Robert & Sutcliffe, Kathleen M., <u>Still Not Safe</u>, Oxford University Press, 2020, p 43.

(92) Webb, Alex, <u>Big Tech's New Vision</u>, Bloomberg Businessweek,December 20, 2021, p.10-11

(93) Webb, Alex, <u>Big Tech's New Vision</u>, Bloomberg Businessweek,December 20, 2021, p.10-11

(94) Wears, R. L., Sutcliffe, K., <u>Still Not Safe</u>, Oxford University Press, 2020., p 216.

(95) Gawande, Atul, <u>The Checklist Manifesto</u>, METROPOLITAN Books Henry Holt and Co., 2009, p 35.

(96) Wears, R. L., Sutcliffe, K., <u>Still Not Safe</u>, Oxford University Press, 2020., p 216

(97) Marx, David, Cal Poly Lecture, January 6, 2022.

(98) Bungay, S., <u>The Art of Action</u>, Nicholas Brealey Publishing, 2011.

(99) Bungay, S., <u>The Art of Action</u>, Nicholas Brealey Publishing, 2011, p 204.

(100) Wears, R. L., Sutcliffe, K., <u>Still Not Safe</u>, Oxford University Press, 2020, p 217-218.

(101) Reason, James, <u>Human Error</u>, Cambridge University Press, 1990, p 241.

(102) Bungay, S., <u>The Art of Action</u>, Nicholas Brealey Publishing, 2011, p 229.

(103) Willink, Jocko & Babin, Leif, <u>Extreme Ownership</u>, St. Martin's Press, 2017.

(104) Sinek, Simon, <u>Leaders Eat Last</u>, Penguin Random House, 2014.

(105) Willink, Jocko & Babin, Leif, <u>Extreme Ownership</u>, St. Martin's Press, 2017.

(106) Sinek, Simon, <u>Leaders Eat Last</u>, Penguin Random House, 2014, p 95.

(107) Bungay, S., <u>The Art of Action</u>, Nicholas Brealey Publishing, 2011, p 229.

(108) Penty, Rebecca & Rocks, David, <u>The WFH Experts in Hot Demand</u>, Bloomberg Businessweek, March 14th, 2022 p.35-36.

(109) Schein, Edgar H., <u>Organizational Culture and Leadership</u>, John Wiley & Sons, Inc., 2017, p 3-5.

(110) Bungay, S., <u>The Art of Action</u>, Nicholas Brealey Publishing, 2011, p 232.

(111) Bungay, S., <u>The Art of Action</u>, Nicholas Brealey Publishing, 2011, p 227-232.

(112) Bungay, S., <u>The Art of Action</u>, Nicholas Brealey Publishing, 2011, p 227-229.

(113) Marx, David, Cal Poly Lecture, January 6, 2022.

(114) Bartleby, <u>Body of Research</u>, The Economist, Feb. 5th 2022. Pg.59

(115) Loehr, James E., <u>Stress for Success</u>, Random House, 1997.

(116) Loehr, James E., <u>Stress for Success</u>, Random House, 1997, p 4.

(117) Loehr, James E., <u>Stress for Success</u>, Random House, 1997.

(118) Loehr, James E., <u>Stress for Success</u>, Random House, 1997, p 56.

(119) Bartleby, <u>Teamwork and the Beatles</u>, The Economist, Dec. 18th 2021, P.53.

(120) Ariely, Dan, <u>Predictably Irrational</u>, Harper Perennial, 2008.pg 175.

(121) Cohen, Arianne, <u>Cancel Meetings to De-Stress Workers</u>, Bloomberg Businessweek, April 4, 2022.pg 35

(122) Willink, Jocko & Babin, Leif, <u>Extreme Ownership</u>, St. Martin's Press, 2017.

(123) Ariely, Dan, <u>Predictably Irrational,</u> Harper Perennial, 2008. pg169-178.

(124) Cohen, Arianne, <u>Improving Hybrid Meetings</u>, Bloomberg Businessweek, April 11, 2022, page, 33.

(125) Heath & Heath, <u>Switch,</u> Broadway Publishing, 2010.

(126) Heath & Heath, <u>Switch,</u> Broadway Publishing, 2010.

(127) Haidt, Jonathen, <u>After Babel</u>, The Atlantic, May 2022. Pg 60.

(128) Haidt, Jonathen, <u>After Babel</u>, The Atlantic, May 2022. Pg 60.

(129) Deal, Terrence, Bolmn, Lee G., <u>Reframing Organizations</u>, John Wiley & Sons, 2008. Pg 69